P9-CRR-235

Orthopaedics
at a Glance

A Handbook of
Disorders, Tests, and
Rehabilitation Strategies

Orthopaedics
at a Glance

A Handbook of
Disorders, Tests, and
Rehabilitation Strategies

Nancy Gann, MS, PT, OCS
Assistant Professor of Physical Therapy
University of Texas Health Science Center at San Antonio
San Antonio, Texas

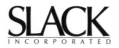

an innovative information, education, and management company

6900 Grove Road • Thorofare, NJ 08086

Copyright © 2001 by SLACK Incorporated

All rights reserved. No part of this book may be reproduced, stored in a retrieval system or transmitted in any form or by any means, electronic, mechanical, photocopying, recording or otherwise, without written permission from the publisher, except for brief quotations embodied in critical articles and reviews.

The author, editor, and publisher cannot accept responsibility for errors or exclusions or for the outcome of the application of the material presented herein. There is no expressed or implied warranty of this book or information imparted by it.

The work SLACK publishes is peer reviewed. Prior to publication, recognized leaders in the field, educators, and clinicians provide important feedback on the concepts and content that we publish. We welcome feedback on this work.

Gann, Nancy.
    Orthopaedics at a glance: a handbook of disorders, tests, and rehabilitation strategies / Nancy Gann.
        p. ; cm.
    Includes bibliographical references and index.
    ISBN 1-55642-500-7 (alk. paper)
        1. Orthopedics--Handbooks, manuals, etc. 2. Musculoskeletal
    system--Diseases--Handbooks, manuals, etc. I. Title.
    [DNLM: 1. Musculoskeletal Diseases--diagnosis--Handbooks. 2. Diagnostic
    Techniques and Procedures--Handbooks. WE 39 G198o 2001]
    RD732.5 .G36 2001
    616.7--dc21

                                                                    00-052217

Printed in the United States of America.
Published by: SLACK Incorporated
                  6900 Grove Road
                  Thorofare, NJ 08086-9447 USA
                  Telephone: 856-848-1000
                  Fax: 856-853-5991
                  www.slackbooks.com

Contact SLACK Incorporated for more information about other books in this field or about the availability of our books from distributors outside the United States.

For permission to reprint material in another publication, contact SLACK Incorporated. Authorization to photocopy items for internal, personal, or academic use is granted by SLACK Incorporated provided that the appropriate fee is paid directly to Copyright Clearance Center. Prior to photocopying items, please contact the Copyright Clearance Center at 222 Rosewood Drive, Danvers, MA 01923 USA; phone: 978-750-8400; website: www.copyright.com; email: info@copyright.com.

For further information on CCC, check CCC Online at the following address: http://www.copyright.com.

Last digit is print number: 10 9 8 7 6 5 4 3 2

CONTENTS

About the Author

Nancy Gann, MS, PT, OCS is assistant professor of physical therapy at the University of Texas Health Science Center at San Antonio, Tex. She holds a bachelor of science degree equivalent in physical therapy from the Mexican Institute of Rehabilitation and an advanced master of science degree in orthopaedic and sports physical therapy from the Institute of Health Professions, Massachusetts General Hospital in Boston, Mass. She is licensed by the state of Texas to practice physical therapy and is certified as an orthopaedic specialist by the American Board of Physical Therapy Specialties.

The author has more than 20 years of experience, having practiced in Mexico City, Boston, New Hampshire, and Texas in a variety of settings and positions, including director of Physical Therapy in hospitals and clinics. In addition to teaching, she has given presentations and has served as a manuscript reviewer, quality assurance consultant, translator, physician advisor, and peer reviewer for a large insurance company.

Nancy is in her eighth year of teaching, with emphasis in orthopaedics and kinesiology. She has published several articles and performed research on ultrasound, one of her main areas of interest, and she is the author of *Orthopaedic Case Studies.*

She currently teaches full-time, performs some clinic work, and continues to be involved in the scholarly activities that enhance the profession.

INTRODUCTION

Orthopaedics at a Glance: A Handbook of Disorders, Tests, and Rehabilitation Strategies was designed for the physical therapy student and clinician and may be useful for physician assistants, primary care physicians, and athletic trainers. Its purpose is to serve as a quick reference for orthopaedic disorders, including characteristics of a diagnosis, its signs and symptoms or examination findings, common special tests, and rehabilitation management.

It is a concise book that should help guide the clinician with basic pathology and treatment in order to deliver effective patient intervention without having to consult large texts. This is a condensed book that assumes the readers are knowledgeable in basic sciences, patient examination and evaluation, and in treatment techniques.

The book is divided into anatomical regions by diagnosis or pathology, starting with the shoulder and ending with the foot and ankle. There are also several special tests, but these do not include those designed to identify muscle tightness, like Thomas' test and Ober's test. Some tests apply to one or more regions, but they have been included only under the most pertinent section. Readers are encouraged to look these tests up in the proximal or distal anatomical regions for the purpose of differential diagnosis. Some tests/treatments not ordinarily performed by therapists have also been included, such as radiology exams, steroid injections, etc. This is not to imply that the non-physician is expected to use these. They are added so that the approaches are more comprehensive. The main goal of this book is to be concise and to serve as a quick reference guide or ancillary text. If more details are needed, the reader is referred to the bibliography.

Some common surgical and postsurgical treatments are also included. They entail brief descriptions and usual treatment approaches to acquaint the clinician with common interventions. Only a few procedures are mentioned because, more often than not, surgical techniques vary from physician to physician, and therefore the treatments are individualized. This obviously applies to nonsurgical approaches as well. Some uncommon pathologies are also included to aid the clinician in differential diagnosis.

As a note, except when not indicated, all interventions include patient education (such as avoidance of aggravators), an individualized home exercise program, and informed consent.

This book also contains a section on radiology with the goal of aiding the clinician in assessing alignment to help manage biomechanical deficits. It is not intended to substitute for the interpretation of a physician or to assume we should practice out of the scope of our profession.

The information contained here is a compilation derived from several sources, as seen in the bibliography. I hope to give credit where credit is due, and I hope this serves as a source of evidence-based practice and stimulates the readers to expand their research interests.

What is presented reflects an eclectic approach to patient management and should not be construed to be the only approach. While the interventions are based on experience and scientific rationale, that is not to say that other strategies may not work, or that every component mentioned in the "treatment box" should be used. Several modalities are outlined, but one should select the least amount of intervention to get the job done right. For example, it is unnecessary to apply iontophoresis and phonophoresis to a patient with posterior tibialis tendinitis, even though both modalities are outlined for this disorder. The choice of which one to use, if any at all, depends on several factors, including availability of equipment and supplies, patient comfort, whether the benefits of ultrasound are needed more than the benefits of electricity, etc. In addition, there are some disorders where, for example, eccentric training is suggested, and while this may be indicated for the athletic population, this may not be advisable for elderly patients.

The treatment choices must be individualized and based on several factors including patient tolerance, previous history, age, occupation, therapist experience, type of rehabilitation setting, stage of the disorder, concomitant problems, availability of resources, etc. Also, one must note that if severe positive findings are not medically addressed first, then physical therapy should not be initiated (positive alar test).

While a few diagnoses may not pertain exclusively to a certain category, they are included for the purpose of aiding in differential diagnosis. An example of this is piriformis syndrome, which anatomically pertains to the hip/buttock region but was placed under the lower back due to its similarity in signs and symptoms in disease processes of spinal origin.

Although the format of this book is user-friendly and categorized in a simple grid format to see the most common aspects of a given disorder, there may be occasions when the patient being treated does not present with all the characteristics mentioned. This is to be expected due to variations in patient population and because there may be coexisting disorders altering a more typical patient presentation. Not all patients who have a bicipital tendinitis will have the exact same signs and symptoms. Therefore, it is important to realize that one cannot "fit" a patient into a box. This is as undesirable as labeling someone "my shoulder patient." Along these same lines, all treatment approaches must be individualized.

The most characteristic aspects of orthopaedic pathology are presented; however, some patients may have too few or several more of the markers outlined and still "qualify" for the approach selected in the clinical decision-making process. This process is applied during the assessment (identifying the problem) and treatment (selecting the best strategy for patient management).

There are several reasons to use this book:
- to confirm one's findings
- to ensure one has performed the most important tests
- to see if there is another sign and/or symptom one should look for
- to determine if one has included all the necessary treatment approaches
- to establish a differential diagnosis
- to refresh one's memory
- to use in class and the clinic

For example, should a patient present with lower extremity numbness, this is an easy reference to help determine the possible sources of the symptoms. By looking under lumbar disorders in the "signs and symptoms" box for the characteristics a patient has, one can see if there is a close match and do a comparison for differential diagnosis. One can then come up with a hypothesis and perform a few special tests to confirm this or rule it out. As the assessment becomes clearer, one has a selection of strategies for appropriate patient management. So, we have at our disposal the most feasible causes of the problem, its typical presentation, special testing procedures for differentiation, and a series of treatment possibilities.

There are some diagnoses listed that are seldom seen by a therapist. They are mentioned, nonetheless, so one knows what they are, what the medical interventions are, and what one might expect to see later if there are any sequelae. More importantly, however, they are included for the purpose of aiding in differential diagnosis and understanding the full picture of the patient's dysfunction.

While the current trend in physical therapy is to use the disablement model, I have chosen not to take that avenue. I share the opinion of Richard Di Fabio, editor in chief of the *Journal of Orthopaedic and Sports Physical Therapy*, when he states that "we should think twice about discarding the pathoanatomical model of disease," as this diminishes the need to discover the source of the patient's problems. I believe that with our knowledge in basic sciences, we are perfectly capable of determining the origin of dysfunction and a logical treatment strategy for the patient's presentation, and this is what is presented in this book.

Nancy Gann, MS, PT, OCS

CHAPTER ONE

SHOULDER DISORDERS, SURGERIES, AND SPECIAL TESTS

TENDINITIS

Characteristics	Signs and Symptoms	Special Tests	Intervention
• Tendon inflammation • Common in the long head of the biceps (LHB), supra-, and infraspinatus tendons. It may be calcific (3% of adults) • Usually due to overuse or trauma • Can lead to tears, degeneration, and impingement • Like most disorders, it can be acute, subacute, or chronic	• Pain with movement • In young patients: pain is from overuse, especially from overhead activities (OHA) • In older patients: the supraspinatus usually undergoes degeneration • Weakness	• Positive empty can test for supraspinatus • Positive impingement signs (Neer and Hawkins) • Positive Speed's test for LHB	• Stop aggravators • Ice massage • Ultrasound (US) • Deep friction massage (DFM) if tolerated • Rotator cuff strengthening • Stretching • No OHA • Joint mobilization and Codman's exercises • Medication

degenerative alteration in a joint cexeessive friction)

———— N O T E S ————

IMPINGEMENT SYNDROME

Characteristics	Signs and Symptoms	Special Tests	Intervention
• Can be structural (spurs) or functional (overuse, especially OHA, tennis, swimming) • Can be primary (without instability) or secondary, due to instability of the glenohumeral joint (GHJ) • The cuff and bursa are pinched against the anterior inferior edge of the acromion and the coracoacromial arch • Usually the supraspinatus is affected at the "critical zone"	• Shoulder pain and referred pain, with upper extremity (UE) weight-bearing and OHA • 3 stages (Neer): 1. <25 years of age, reversible, painful arc, decreased range of movement (ROM), and edema, tender to palpate 2. 25- to 40-year-olds with fibrosis, nonreversible by modification of activity, soft tissue crepitus 3. >40 years of age, spur and tear, atrophy of the infraspinatus; LHB can be involved; weakness	• Hypo- or hypermobility • Painful arc • Positive impingement sign • Positive supraspinatus test • Tenderness to palpation • Decreased joint space on radiographs • Shoulder girdle muscle imbalances	• See tendinitis • Levator scapula stretches • Joint mobilizations: posterior and inferior glides (PG and IG) if not hypermobile • Pain-free cuff and scapular strengthening • Surgery: arthroscopic subacromial decompression or acromioplasty

--------- N O T E S ---------

Other shoulder problems arise from forceful muscle contractions (external rotation [ER], internal rotation [IR], and LHB), contusions (linebacker's arm or blocker's exostosis), neural damage from traction injuries or direct blows, overstretch injuries of muscles in different positions (shoulder flexion with elbow extension), subluxation of the LHB, throwing injuries, epiphyseal and avulsion fractures (little leaguer's shoulder), sympathetic problems like shoulder-hand syndrome, postural faults (kyphosis), myofascial pain syndrome (MFPS), etc.

ROTATOR CUFF TEARS

Characteristics	Signs and Symptoms	Special Tests	Intervention
• Can be due to degeneration, trauma, overuse (OHA), or vascular problems • Usually in men older than 40 • Can be complete or partial • Grade I: small tear if <1 cm • Grade II: medium tear if >1cm but <5 cm • Grade III: massive tear if >5 cm	• Deep ache • Referred pain • Decreased ROM, especially abduction • Rotator cuff weakness • Atrophy • Scapular substitutions/hypomobility • Altered scapulothoracic rhythm	• Positive drop arm test • Positive empty can test • Positive impingement sign • If the tear is in biceps: positive Speed's, positive Yergason's, and Ludington's last two tests (not included) • Difficulty with abduction • Shoulder hiking if ER is weak	• Grades I and II: rest, ice, maintain ROM • Stop aggravators • Gradually strengthen rotators, then abductors • Caution with IG • Address scapulothoracic joint • Others: repair and decompression

— N O T E S —

GLENOHUMERAL JOINT INSTABILITY

Characteristics	Signs and Symptoms	Special Tests	Intervention
• 3 basic types: 1. Multi-directional (MDI) 2. Traumatic, unidirectional with Bankart lesion requiring surgery (TUBS) 3. Traumatic, multidirectional, bilateral, requiring rehabilitation or inferior capsular shift (AMBRI)	• Hypermobility • May or may not be painful • Weakness • Atrophy • Clicking • Decreased function • May lead to dislocation	• Positive sulcus sign • Positive apprehension test • Positive load and shift tests • May have a positive clunk test if the labrum is torn • Other instability tests may also be positive	• Strengthen IR, cuff, adductors, and scapular muscles • Scapular stabilization • Restore muscle balance (force couples) • Avoid ER, abduction (abd), and hyperextension • Proprioceptive neuromuscular facilitation (PNF), motor control, and closed kinetic chain exercises

ACUTE BURSITIS

Characteristics	Signs and Symptoms	Special Tests	Intervention
• Rare but can occur with activities like swimming • May be due to calcific tendinitis or trauma • Pain builds over 12 to 72 hours • Often self-limiting	• Referred lateral arm pain • All motions are painful • May have history of chronic tendinitis • Active range of motion (AROM) restricted in all planes	• Passive range of motion (PROM) restricted in noncapsular pattern • Empty end-feel • Palpation: warm and tender	• Medication • Ice • Sling • Codman's exercises • Grades I and II mobilizations • Nonthermal US

ANTERIOR DISLOCATION

Characteristics	Signs and Symptoms	Special Tests	Intervention
• 95% of GHJ dislocations are anterior • Can be subcoracoid (most common), subglenoid, subclavicular, or subspinous and may be recurrent (92% rate in people <20 years of age) • Usually due to trauma in ER and abduction • Usually damages the anterior capsule, the labrum, the subscapularis, and the rotator cuff	• Results in instability • Hypermobility • Weakness • Hill-Sachs lesion • Bankart lesion in 85% of dislocations (labrum and anterior capsule/ligament disruption) • Atrophy • Pain • Clicking • Some people do this voluntarily	• Positive anterior drawer test • Positive anterior apprehension test • Positive clunk test • Positive load and shift test • Other anterior instability tests may also be positive	• Closed reduction and sling (immobilization time is longer for younger patients) • Avoid ER, abduction, and hyperextension • No anterior glides or OHA • Strengthen IR, ER, and adductors • Pliometrics, closed chain, and PNF exercises • Surgery: opened or closed anterior capsular shift

---

N O T E S

SLAP Lesions (Superior Labrum, Anterior and Posterior)

Characteristics	Signs and Symptoms	Special Tests	Intervention
• Tear of the long head of the biceps tendon anchor/superior labral complex • Usually due to a FOOSH injury (falling on the outstretched hand) or gymnastics (on rings) • These lesions accompany 16% to 31% of cuff tears	• Pain, especially with OHA • Painful catching and popping • Weakness in abduction and flexion • Does not necessarily have instability • Four types: superior labral fraying, fraying and stripping of labrum and biceps, bucket-handle tear of labrum, and bucket-handle tear with biceps tear	• Magnetic resonance imaging (MRI) • Positive Speed's test • Positive superior labral tear test • Positive SLAP-prehension test • Differentiate between acromioclavicular joint (ACJ) and Bankart lesion	• Conservative treatment for a few weeks if the shoulder is functional, similar to rotator cuff tears • Postsurgical approach is similar to Bankart repair, but avoid external rotation beyond 0 degrees for 3 weeks

---

N O T E S

ACROMIOCLAVICULAR SEPARATION

Characteristics	Signs and Symptoms	Special Tests	Intervention
• Usually due to a FOOSH injury or a fall on the shoulder tip • Acromioclavicular (AC) ligament is overstretched • Grades: I: pain, no instability II: AC ligament and capsular tear, pain, swelling, laxity III: AC and coracoclavicular (CC) tear and instability	• Shoulder tip pain • Complete separation results in "shoulder pointer" or a bump on the shoulder • Step deformity	• Positive AC shear test • X-ray (normal AC space is 2 to 5 mm wide; normal CC space is 1.1 to 1.3 mm wide)	• Acute stage: immobilization • Sling for 2 weeks • ROM exercises • Codman's exercises • Strengthening • May need surgery if grade III

PROXIMAL HUMERUS FRACTURES

Characteristics	Signs and Symptoms	Special Tests	Intervention
• Common in older patients • Usually with swelling and bruising • Can result in capsulitis • Can be two-part, three-part, or four-part fracture • Surgery if completely displaced	• Sharp pain at the shoulder • Referred pain • Decreased ROM • Weakness • Atrophy • Hypomobility • Tissue texture abnormalities	• X-ray	• If stable, gentle PROM after 3 days • Codman's exercises • Early AROM • Submaximal isometrics • Tubing exercises at 4 to 6 weeks • Scapulothoracic and GHJ mobilizations

ADHESIVE CAPSULITIS (FROZEN SHOULDER)

Characteristics	Signs and Symptoms	Special Tests	Intervention
• Can be primary or idiopathic and secondary, due to immobilization, reflex sympathetic dystrophy (RSD), chest surgery, kyphosis • Insidious onset • Has three stages: freezing, frozen, and thawing • More common in middle-aged women	• Decreased ROM • If acute: pain radiating to elbow, night pain, and pain with PROM • If chronic, pain decreases and is more localized; stiffness and atrophy persist • Insulin-dependent diabetic patients also acquire this but with a different capsular pattern (IR>ER>ABD)	• Capsular pattern (ER>ABD>IR) • PROM limited by pain, guarding, and capsular end feel • Decreased joint mobility, especially IG	• US (for heat) • DFM if tolerated • Joint mobilizations • PROM and stretching (increase ER then abduction) • Scapulothoracic mobilizations • Pulleys • Contract-relax • Strengthening • Functional exercises

———— N O T E S ————

ROTATOR CUFF REPAIR

Characteristics	Signs and Symptoms	Special Tests	Intervention
• Acromioplasty (decompression, debridement, and excision of acromion) • Arthroscopic surgery (sub-acromial decompression) • Arthroscopically assisted repair • Tendon transfers	• Depending on the technique, the patient may be restricted in active ER for 4 weeks, especially if the tear is massive	• Surgical	• Based on doctor (MD) • Modalities as needed for pain and inflammation • Abduction pillow or sling • Wrist/hand/elbow exercises • Passive flexion, progressing to active assistive (A/A), Codman's, and when tissues have healed, cuff strengthening exercises • Scapular mobilizations/stabilization • Pulley exercises

———— N O T E S ————

BANKART REPAIR

Characteristics	Signs and Symptoms	Special Tests	Intervention
• Reattachment to the glenoid rim of the avulsed anterior GH capsuloligamentous structures including the labrum if damaged • Anterior capsulorrhaphy, shifting the capsule to the labrum • May be done arthroscopically or opened (if labrum is frayed) • The deltoid may be split or detached	• The patient may be restricted in active ER for 4 weeks and may never regain full motion, which is one of the purposes of the surgery	• Surgical	• As in previous table, progressing to A/A in flexion in supine only to 120 degrees and ER at 20 degrees of abduction to a max of 20 degrees and IR to 45 degrees; submaximal isometrics • At 3 to 4 weeks: progress to 140 degrees flexion, 20 degrees ER at 45 degrees abduction, and IR to max of 60 degrees; scapular strengthening • At 8 to 10 weeks: progress to full ROM (except ER)

——————— N O T E S ———————

SPECIAL TESTS

SUPRASPINATUS TEST

Purpose	Positive Test	Interpretation	Comments
• To test for the integrity of the tendon • May be present with subacromial bursitis and incomplete tears	• Pain and/or weakness ensue during downward pressure on the flexed (90 degrees), abducted, and internally rotated shoulder (scaption)	• Supraspinatus tendon is inflamed or torn • Compare with arm flexed in neutral	• May be accompanied by positive drop arm test, Speed's test, and impingement sign • Full can test is also accurate, especially for weakness • Also called empty can test

IMPINGEMENT SIGN (NEER)

Purpose	Positive Test	Interpretation	Comments
• To pinch the LHB or the supraspinatus tendon between the head of the humerus and the acromion	• Superior glenohumeral joint pain appears as the shoulder is placed into elevation with over-pressure	• Indicates overuse of the tendon(s)	• See above • May be combined with internal rotation with adduction at 90 degrees of flexion (Hawkins test)

SPEED'S TEST

Purpose	Positive Test	Interpretation	Comments
• To test for irritation of the LHB • May be positive if there is a SLAP lesion	• Pain arises when resistance is applied to the flexed (90 degrees) and externally rotated shoulder, with elbow extended and supinated	• Indicates tendinitis or fraying of the LHB	• May be accompanied by impingement sign and supraspinatus test

DROP ARM TEST

Purpose	Positive Test	Interpretation	Comments
• To test the integrity of the rotator cuff muscles	• There is an inability to actively descend the abducted shoulder (weakness)	• Rotator cuff is torn	• May present with atrophy, abductor weakness, and scapular substitutions • Also called Codman's sign

PAINFUL ARC

Purpose	Positive Test	Interpretation	Comments
• To determine whether there is an impingement	• Pain while actively abducting the arm, usually between 45 to 60 degrees and 120 degrees	• Impingement is present	• If painful at end range, the AC joint may be involved

LOAD AND SHIFT TEST

Purpose	Positive Test	Interpretation	Comments
• To determine the integrity of the anterior glenohumeral structures • Assesses hypermobility/instability	• Excessive anterior displacement or pain when passively compressing the humeral head in the glenoid and translating it forward	• Indicates hypermobility/joint instability • Has three grades • Compare to other side	• A 25% translation can be normal • Can be used also for posterior translation

SUPERIOR LABRAL TEAR TEST

Purpose	Positive Test	Interpretation	Comments
• To determine if there is a SLAP lesion • This test is 100% sensitive and 90% specific for type II SLAP lesions (especially for the superior labrum)	• The patient sits and abducts the shoulder to 90 degrees; externally rotate the arm in maximum pronation and maximum supination with the elbow flexed	• The test is positive if pain is provoked only in pronation or if this position is more painful than supination • It may identify tenosynovitis	• This test places the shoulder in an apprehension position • Tension of the LHB increases when the forearm is pronated

SLAPPREHENSION TEST

Purpose	Positive Test	Interpretation	Comments
• To determine if there is a SLAP lesion • This test is 87% sensitive for unstable SLAP lesions	• The patient performs horizontal adduction and internal rotation with elbow extension. The test is then repeated with the arm in external rotation	• The test is positive if there is apprehension, pain in the biceps groove, and an audible or palpable click while in IR, which then decreases with ER	• Elbow extension and shoulder IR places traction on the long head of the biceps • Need to differentiate with impingement and ACJ arthrosis

CLUNK TEST

Purpose	Positive Test	Interpretation	Comments
• To determine the integrity of the capsular labrum • A Bankart lesion is a tear in the anterior inferior labrum and a SLAP lesion is in the superior, anterior, and posterior labrum	• A clunk is heard or felt when the patient is supine and the arm is fully abducted; place one hand on the posterior aspect of the head of the humerus, while the other hand holds the arm above the elbow. The first hand pushes anteriorly while the other hand rotates the humerus laterally	• A "clunk" indicates a labrum tear, usually anteriorly	• This test may cause apprehension if there is anterior instability, so it must be done with care

IMPINGEMENT RELIEF TEST

Purpose	Positive Test	Interpretation	Comments
• To see if there is an impingement	• Perform an IG during active abduction	• Pain is relieved during the glide	• Should be done for painful arcs

APPREHENSION TEST

Purpose	Positive Test	Interpretation	Comments
• To test for anterior shoulder instability	• The patient has a feeling of apprehension like the shoulder will dislocate upon placing the joint in slow abduction and external rotation • Must be done carefully, usually in supine	• This means the shoulder is unstable	• Can also be performed with the arm horizontally adducted and internally rotated while in 90 degrees of flexion to test for posterior instability • Also called crank test

FEAGIN TEST

Purpose	Positive Test	Interpretation	Comments
• To determine the presence of anterior and inferior instability	• There is apprehension and increased inferior motion while the arm is pushed down when abducted and anchored on the examiner's shoulder	• There is anterior and inferior instability and laxity of the inferior glenohumeral ligament	• This test is a modification of the sulcus sign in which there is a dip in the joint with downward traction, while the arm is at the side

SULCUS SIGN

Purpose	Positive Test	Interpretation	Comments
• To see if there is inferior instability	• Pull the relaxed arm distally by the elbow	• A dip at the GHJ indicates laxity	• The wider the sulcus, the worse the condition

LEFFERT'S TEST

Purpose	Positive Test	Interpretation	Comments
• To determine the presence of anterior and inferior instability	• Index is on head of the humerus, midfinger on coracoid process, and thumb on posterior side. Abduct and externally rotate the arm. If the index translates forward, the test is positive	• The examiner's fingers return to the same plane when the arm is brought back to neutral	• Also called anterior instability test • The patient is supine

ACROMIOCLAVICULAR SHEAR TEST

Purpose	Positive Test	Interpretation	Comments
• To determine if there is an AC joint pathology	• Cup your hands over the deltoid, covering the clavicle and the spine of the scapula, and squeeze the heels of your hands together. If positive, there will be pain and/or abnormal motion	• May indicate a ligamentous disruption	• This test is done with the patient sitting

CHAPTER TWO

ELBOW DISORDERS
AND
SPECIAL TESTS

LATERAL EPICONDYLITIS (TENNIS ELBOW)

Characteristics	Signs and Symptoms	Special Tests	Intervention
• May be due to a highstrung tennis racket or gripping the racket too tightly, from gardening, other repetitive motions, or trauma • Common at age 35 and older • Usually occurs after repeated and/or forceful wrist extension • Usually involves the extensor carpi radialis brevis (ECRB) due to overuse • Onset is usually gradual	• Pain and tenderness on lateral epicondyle and extensor muscles • May radiate to posterior forearm • Pain with passive wrist extensor stretching and with resistance • Morning stiffness	• Positive tennis elbow or Cozen's test • Reproduction of symptoms with previous maneuvers • History of overuse or trauma	• Limit repetitive motion • Cock-up splint and/or forearm cuff • Ice massage • US, phono- or iontophoresis • DFM if tolerated • Gentle wrist extensor stretches • Low level strengthening when symptoms decrease

Note: There is also posterior tennis elbow, which is triceps tendinitis due to throwing.

———————— N O T E S ————————

MEDIAL EPICONDYLITIS			
Characteristics	*Signs and Symptoms*	*Special Tests*	*Intervention*
• "Golfer's elbow" • Less common than lateral epicondylitis • Can occur in expert tennis players • Can cause ulnar nerve compression	• Pain over medial epicondyle, pronator teres, and/or flexor carpi radialis (FCR)	• History of overuse • Pain with resisted pronation	• Similar to tennis elbow but with gentle wrist flexor stretches

BURSITIS			
Characteristics	*Signs and Symptoms*	*Special Tests*	*Intervention*
• Inflammation of the olecranon bursae • Common in students ("student's elbow") • Usually due to prolonged leaning, but also due to trauma, infection, and gout	• Thickened bursae • Tenderness • May have a callus • Pain with ROM • Elbow extension may be slightly limited	• Nonspecific tenderness • Observation	• Ice or heat • US • Phono- or iontophoresis • Protective padding • Decrease the pressure

— N O T E S —

RHEUMATOID ARTHRITIS

Characteristics	Signs and Symptoms	Special Tests	Intervention
• Autoimmune inflammatory disease • Can involve one or both elbows and other joints • Can cause instability	• Pain, especially at radiohumeral joint (RHJ) • Swelling • Increased local temperature • Decreased ROM and function	• Blood test • X-ray • Positive valgus and/or varus tests	• Medication • Rest and ice • Gentle ROM • Assistive devices • Joint protection

FRACTURES

Characteristics	Signs and Symptoms	Special Tests	Intervention
• Common in children and teens due to epiphyseal plates not fully closed • Common ones: supracondylar, head of the radius, olecranon process, and medial epicondyle • Often associated with dislocations • Common with FOOSH injuries and direct blows • Can result in Volkman's ischemia	• Pain • Deformation • Minimal to no AROM • Swelling • Unwillingness to move the arm	• X-ray • Mechanism of injury • Patient's age • Observation in some cases	• Immobilization or surgery • When healed: heat, whirlpool, massage, ROM, stretching, and strengthening, progressing to functional exercises

Note: Monteggia's, Galeazzi's, Essex-Lopresti are some common types of elbow fractures/dislocations.

LITTLE LEAGUE ELBOW

Characteristics	Signs and Symptoms	Special Tests	Intervention
• Avulsion stress fracture of the medial epicondyle due to repetitive motion: throwing during the acceleration phase with forceful forearm flexion with valgus • Seen in children and teenagers • Has three grades; grade III is more than 5 mm separation of the epiphysis	• Progressive pain • Tenderness • Decreased ROM (>15 degrees) • Decreased throwing distance • Can result in osteochondritis of the capitellum, avascular necrosis of the radial head, and loose bodies	• X-ray • History • Positive valgus test	• Rest • Stop playing • Immobilization • When healed, treatment is similar to fractures with gradual progression to sports • Surgery if advanced

—————— N O T E S ——————

OSTEOCHONDRITIS DISSECANS

Characteristics	Signs and Symptoms	Special Tests	Intervention
• Avascularity of subchondral bone • Bone separates from articular cartilage like a fracture (capitellum) • Idiopathic, in 10-year-olds and teenagers (Panner's disease) • Frequent in compression injuries, especially gymnastics (FOOSH)	• May have a mild flexion contracture • Throwing problems • Pain, especially with UE weight-bearing	• X-ray • History	• Rest and ice • When healed, stretching and strengthening exercises • Sports modification • Return to sports when function is restored without pain • Surgery if loose bodies are present

— N O T E S —

VOLKMAN'S ISCHEMIC CONTRACTURE

Characteristics	Signs and Symptoms	Special Tests	Intervention
• Acute arterial obstruction causing infarction of muscles in the forearm • Most common after supracondylar fractures of the humerus and with tight casts • After 6 hours, the muscle can become necrotic, eventually scar, and develop into a flexion contracture	• Pain in forearm flexors and with passive finger extension • Absent radial pulse • Edema, pallor, decreased sensation, coldness, paresthesias, paralysis, and clawing	• Palpation, observation, and history • PROM limitation • Based on signs and symptoms	• Requires immediate medical attention • Release cast • Extend the elbow • Massage • Whirlpool • Electrical stimulation (ES) to damaged muscles • Surgery

———— N O T E S ————

ULNAR NERVE COMPRESSION

Characteristics	Signs and Symptoms	Special Tests	Intervention
• Nerve entrapment • Usually due to prolonged elbow flexion, overuse (eg, musicians, pitchers), increased valgus (medial instability), trauma (fracture of the medial epicondyle), muscular compression (hypertrophy of elbow extensors or flexor carpi ulnaris [FCU]), or degenerative changes (spurs)	• Decreased power grip and key pinch • Weakness • Elbow and forearm pain • Aching • Paresthesias of the last two fingers • Atrophy • Symptoms appear while reading or at night if originating at the elbow	• Positive Tinel's sign • Positive upper limb tension test (ULTT) • Positive Froment's sign (adductor pollicis) • Positive elbow flexion test • Positive nerve conduction velocity (NCV) tests	• Rest • Avoid aggravators • Gentle upper limb tension stretching • Phonophoresis or ES • Splint in elbow extension, especially at night • Maintain ROM and strength • Surgery if severe (decompression or transposition) • After surgery: protection, ROM, splinting, progress to motor retraining and desensitization

Note: Called cubital tunnel syndrome at the elbow and guyon canal compression at the wrist.

———————— N O T E S ————————

RADIAL NERVE COMPRESSION

Characteristics	Signs and Symptoms	Special Tests	Intervention
• Nerve entrapment • Compression under the ECRB, arcade of Frohse, between the supinator muscle and the radial head, between the ECRL and the brachioradialis tendons or axilla • Also called radial tunnel syndrome • Called Wartenberg's syndrome if compressed between the extensor carpi radialis longus (ECRL) and brachioradialis • Can be due to trauma, repetitive supination, pronation, or wrist extension	• Decreased wrist and metacarpal phalangeal (MCP) extension • Weakness is uncommon • Diffuse pain 5 cm distal to lateral epicondyle in which there is tenderness to palpation • Aching • Paresthesias • Usually no true sensory abnormalities • Interphalangeal (IP) joint extension can be full due to intrinsic activity • May have radiating pain	• Easily confused with tennis elbow • Pain with resistance to ECRB • Positive Tinel's sign • Positive ULTT • Resisted supination with wrist flexion and elbow extension can reproduce the pain • Positive NCV test	• Avoid aggravators • Rest • Medication • Splint for 3 to 6 months, avoiding pressure at the level of the entrapment • Phonophoresis or ES • Maintain ROM and strength

Note: Also known as posterior interosseous syndrome (PIS), superficial radial nerve entrapment, "Saturday Night" or crutch palsy.

MEDIAN NERVE COMPRESSION

Characteristics	Signs and Symptoms	Special Tests	Intervention
• Nerve entrapment • Common after fracture of the elbow, especially in children; also due to pronator teres hypertrophy or compression between the two heads of pronator teres, tight casts, or from the ligament of Struthers • Can be due to crush injuries or overuse, especially with pronation and gripping	• Decreased opposition • Flat thenar eminence • Weakness, especially APB • Insidious anterior forearm pain • Aching • Paresthesias • Atrophy • No sensory changes with AIS	• Positive Phalen's test • Pronation aggravates the symptoms • Positive Tinel's sign • Positive ULTT • Positive "tear drop" pinch with AIS • Resisted pronation with elbow flexion causes pain • Positive NCV test	• See previous treatment • Splint, especially at night • Phonophoresis • ES • Maintain ROM and strength • Surgery

Note: Also known as carpal tunnel syndrome at the wrist, pronator syndrome, and anterior interosseous syndrome (AIS) at the forearm.

--- N O T E S ---

SPECIAL TESTS

LIGAMENTOUS INSTABILITY TEST

Purpose	Positive Test	Interpretation	Comments
• To determine the integrity of collateral ligaments of the elbow	• There is pain and/or laxity on the medial side when a valgus force is applied to the flexed elbow (25 degrees)	• Indicates there is a sprain or tear of the ligament	• Also performed on the lateral side with a varus force • Called valgus or varus tests

LATERAL EPICONDYLITIS TEST

Purpose	Positive Test	Interpretation	Comments
• To determine if there is lateral epicondylitis or tennis elbow	• Pain at the wrist extensor origin with resisted wrist extension	• Indicates inflammation or tearing at the tendinous junction of the extensors	• May also present as weakness • Also known as Cozen's test

MEDIAL EPICONDYLITIS TEST

Purpose	Positive Test	Interpretation	Comments
• To determine if there is flexor/pronator tendinitis	• Pain over the medial epicondyle with resistance to wrist and elbow flexion while in elbow flexion and supination	• Indicates inflammation or tearing at the tendinous junction of the flexors	• May also present with a weak grip • Also known as golfer's elbow test

ELBOW FLEXION TEST

Purpose	Positive Test	Interpretation	Comments
• To determine if the ulnar nerve is compressed at the level of the elbow	• Paresthesias on the ulnar nerve distribution upon maintaining full elbow flexion for 1 to 3 minutes	• Indicates cubital tunnel syndrome	• Symptoms should gradually decrease with elbow extension

TINEL'S SIGN

Purpose	Positive Test	Interpretation	Comments
• To determine if there is neuritis • This test may be performed on several areas of the forearm at the level of an entrapment	• Tingling and/or pain ensue with tapping between the olecranon and the medial epicondyle and between the olecranon and the lateral epicondyle	• If present on the lateral side, it indicates superficial radial nerve involvement; and if on the medial side, it indicates ulnar nerve compromise	• Tingling means there is regeneration • Pain and tingling means there is injury and degeneration • Can be present in 24% of the normal population

——————— N O T E S ———————

CHAPTER THREE

WRIST AND HAND DISORDERS AND SPECIAL TESTS

SPRAINS

Characteristics	Signs and Symptoms	Special Tests	Intervention
• Traumatic onset, usually due to FOOSH injuries or axial loading • Can be up to 3 degrees, according to severity	• Localized pain • Pain increases with motion • Limited function • Decreased weight-bearing ability of the upper extremity	• End ROM can reproduce the symptoms • Tenderness over the affected joint • Positive valgus or varus tests	• Anti-inflammatories • PRICE if acute (protection, rest, ice, compression, and elevation) • US, DFM • Progress to gradual ROM, strengthening, and functional activities

COLLES' FRACTURE

Characteristics	Signs and Symptoms	Special Tests	Intervention
• Distal radius fracture with radial deviation of the distal segment • Ulnar styloid can avulse • Common after menopause • Usually due to FOOSH injuries • Some complications include RSD, carpal tunnel syndrome (CTS), nonunion, and deformity	• "Dinner-fork" deformity: distal fragment is angulated dorsally • Smith's fracture: distal fragment is in a palmar direction	• If displaced, there is deformity • X-ray • Some fractures are now being treated with an injection of calcium phosphate paste, which is later replaced by bone. Motion can start in 2 weeks	• Reduction of the fracture (opened or closed) and immobilization for 4 to 8 weeks • Splint • Edema control • ROM exercises • Mobilizations if hypomobile after healing • Strengthening • Functional activities

DE QUERVAIN'S TENOSYNOVITIS

Characteristics	Signs and Symptoms	Special Tests	Intervention
• Inflammation of the synovial lining of the abductor pollicis longus (APL) and extensor pollicis brevis (EPB) sheath, leading to stenosis • Insidious onset, such as from pinching or wringing out clothes with wrist in ulnar deviation (UD) • May also occur due to edema/hormones from pregnancy	• Pain with wringing and grasping • Pain can radiate into the thumb and the distal forearm (radial aspect) • Tenderness over the radial styloid process	• Pain is reproduced with resisted thumb extension and abduction • Positive Finkelstein's test	• Avoid aggravators • PRICE • Phono- or iontophoresis • ES • DFM • Tendon gliding • Tenosynovectomy

— N O T E S —

REFLEX SYMPATHETIC DYSTROPHY SYNDROME

Characteristics	Signs and Symptoms	Special Tests	Intervention
• Unknown etiology	• Hyperalgesia (pain disproportionate to the lesion)	• Observation: swelling and vasomotor instability	• Desensitization
• Common complication of Colles' fractures	• Capsular tightness/stiffness	• History	• Joint loading
• Can include causalgia, Sudek's atrophy, shoulder-hand syndrome	• Hyperhydrosis	• X-ray	• AROM
	• Vasoconstriction in later stages	• Stellate ganglion block	• ES, US, massage, and paraffin
• Three stages: acute (1 to 3 months), dystrophic (3 to 6 or 9 months), and atrophic	• Atrophy		• Splints
	• Trophic changes (skin is thin and glossy, hands are clammy, and nails are brittle)		• Medications to inhibit the sympathetic function
• Abnormal sympathetic reflex	• Osteoporosis		• Contrast baths
• Some patients have certain psychic traits: insecure, low pain threshold, depression	• Edema		• Sympathectomy
• Can cause stiff hand syndrome			• Stellate ganglion block
• Can occur in 5% of traumatic injuries			

Note: RSD is also called complex regional pain syndrome; type I: similar to RSD, tissue damage with no nerve damage; type II: with nerve damage.

CARPAL TUNNEL SYNDROME

Characteristics	Signs and Symptoms	Special Tests	Intervention
• Increased pressure in the carpal tunnel • More common in women • Affects the median nerve • More insidious than traumatic: due to vibration, direct pressure, repetitive motion, prolonged gripping, pinching, or wrist flexion • May come with double-crush injury, so the neck may be involved • May occur during pregnancy	• Paresthesias on the first three to four fingers • Symptoms increase at night • Decreased fine motor skills • Burning • Pain that may or may not radiate • Weakness of abductor pollicis brevis • Thenar atrophy	• Electromyelogram (EMG)/NCV • Positive Tinel's sign • Positive Phalen's maneuver • Vibration test • Semmes Weinstein filament test • Two-point discrimination test • Square-shaped wrist • Screen the cervical area • Positive flexion/compression test	• Avoid aggravators, job modification • Tendon gliding exercises • Tunnel stretching • Splint, especially at night • Glove/pad • Phonophoresis • ES • Steroid injections or surgery

——————— N O T E S ———————

WARTENBERG'S SYNDROME

Characteristics	Signs and Symptoms	Special Tests	Intervention
• Superficial radial nerve entrapment or neuritis between the tendons of the ECRL and brachioradialis at wrist level (from tight watch) • See radial nerve entrapment (elbow) • Also known as cheiralgia paresthetica • Not very common	• Paresthesias on the dorsal aspect of the first web space • Pain • No overt sensory changes • Weakness is uncommon	• Positive Tinel's sign at the site of the compression • Reproduction of symptoms with elbow extension, pronation, and wrist flexion	• Avoid aggravators • Phonophoresis or ES • Splint for 3 to 6 months, avoiding pressure at the level of the entrapment • Neurolysis

DUPUYTREN'S CONTRACTURE

Characteristics	Signs and Symptoms	Special Tests	Intervention
• Thickening of the palmar fascia of the finger flexors or the thumb • Unknown etiology but suspected to be genetic (European descent), due to repeated trauma or vascular changes • More common in men between the ages of 50 and 70 than women • May be associated with diabetes	• MCP and/or proximal interphalangeal (PIP) flexion contracture of the fourth and/or fifth fingers • Decreased function • Usually not painful	• Observation: MCP unable to fully extend, and there is palpable thickening	• Conservative treatment is not very successful: US, iontophoresis, very gentle stretching • Local injections • Surgery in some cases

GAMEKEEPER'S THUMB (SKIER'S THUMB)

Characteristics	Signs and Symptoms	Special Tests	Intervention
• Sprain or rupture of the ulnar collateral ligament of the thumb (MCP) • Can avulse in adolescents • Occurs due to extreme thumb abduction	• Tenderness over the ulnar ligament and joint • Instability at the MCP joint • Decreased function	• History • Palpation • Positive valgus stress test	• Immobilization in short-arm spica for 6 weeks • ROM and strengthening after immobilization • May need surgery if volar plate is injured

MALLET FINGER

Characteristics	Signs and Symptoms	Special Tests	Intervention
• Avulsion of the extensor digitorum communis (EDC) or extensor pollicis longus (EPL) tendon from the base of the distal interphalangeal (DIP) joint, usually from catching a ball incorrectly • Lack of DIP extension • Heals in 6 to 12 months	• DIP remains flexed • Pain • Decreased function	• During active extension, the DIP stays flexed	• Splint with DIP in neutral or extension and PIP in flexion or free for 6 weeks • Gentle active flexion and extension after 6 to 8 weeks

POSITIVE OR NEGATIVE ULNAR VARIANCE

Characteristics	Signs and Symptoms	Special Tests	Intervention
• Ulnar variance is the relative length of the ulna compared to the radius • Neutral variance is present when both surfaces are even • Positive variance: long ulna; can cause degeneration and perforation of the triangular fibrocartilaginous complex (TFCC), wear and tear of the carpals, growth inhibition of radius, and ulnar impaction syndrome • Negative variance: short ulna; can predispose to Kienböck's disease • Not very common but can be seen in gymnasts	• Pain, especially with weight-bearing at the wrist, with extension, pronation, and supination • If negative variance, pain is in the "snuffbox" area • Pronation can appear to increase the variance and supination can appear to decrease it	• X-ray • For positive variance, compress the wrist and ulnarly deviate it to reproduce the symptoms	• Decrease loads • Ulnar gutter splint • Surgery if conservative measures fail: 6 weeks of immobilization conservatively and/or postoperatively • Postoperative approach is geared mainly at reestablishing function

KIENBÖCK'S DISEASE

Characteristics	Signs and Symptoms	Special Tests	Intervention
• Avascular necrosis of the lunate (lunatomalacia), usually after a fracture • Unknown etiology (trauma, heavy labor) • More common in men 2:1, 20 to 40 years of age • Four stages (radiographic) • Associated with negative variance	• Pain with motion and after activity • Tenderness over the lunate • Decreased ROM and grip strength • Prominent lunate with hyperflexion	• X-ray (lunate squeezed between radius and capitate during loading) • Positive finger extension test	• Stage I focuses on pain control and increasing grip • Prolonged casting • Surgery for other stages (grafts, pins, osteotomy, arthroplasty)

LUNATE DISLOCATION

Characteristics	Signs and Symptoms	Special Tests	Intervention
• Most frequent carpal dislocation but uncommon • Difficult to diagnose • Usually from hyperextension of the wrist (FOOSH) • Usually dislocates palmarly (unless fall was in flexion) • Can cause CTS	• Localized pain • Tenderness to palpation • Localized swelling • Ligamentous laxity • May have hypermobility • May cause paresthesias if median nerve is involved	• X-ray (multiple views, lunate appears palmarly flexed) • Positive Murphy's sign	• Opened or closed reduction and immobilization for 6 to 8 weeks • Postimmobilization treatment is geared toward increasing ROM, function, and strength

PISIFORM OR HAMATE HOOK FRACTURE

Characteristics	Signs and Symptoms	Special Tests	Intervention
• Due to FOOSH injury or a blow from the handle of a racket or club • Other fractures include boxer's and Bennett's at the metacarpals, usually from punching	• Pain over the fracture site • May cause paresthesias if ulnar nerve is involved (Guyon's canal)	• X-ray • History	• Immobilization • Surgery • ROM and strengthening after healing to restore function

SCAPHOID FRACTURE

Characteristics	Signs and Symptoms	Special Tests	Intervention
• Difficult to diagnose • Healing times range from 5 to 20 weeks due to poor blood flow • Most occur at the waist of the bone and heal after 12 weeks • Can occur due to falls on the wrist in extension, especially in 12- to 15-year-olds	• History • Local pain and swelling in anatomical snuffbox • Can cause complications later in life, such as degenerative joint disease, instability, or lead to necrosis	• X-ray • History • Local pain and swelling	• Immobilization in a thumb spica cast for up to 12 weeks • Surgery (open reduction internal fixation [ORIF]) • Postimmobilization: edema control, ROM, and strengthening exercises progressing as tolerated

INSTABILITIES (DISI AND VISI)

Characteristics	Signs and Symptoms	Special Tests	Intervention
• Scapholunate instability (due to FOOSH) leads to dorsal intercalated segmental instability (DISI) (lunate tilts dorsally) • Triquetrolunate instability (less common) leads to volar intercalated segmental instability (VISI)	• Pain • Decreased grip strength • Decreased ROM • Tenderness and laxity • Need to differentiate this from wrist sprains in which there is less hypermobility	• X-ray (Terry Thomas > 2 mm sign) • Positive finger extension test	• Surgery (pinning) • Postsurgical approach: edema control, ROM, and strengthening exercises progressing as tolerated

Note: There is also midcarpal instability on proximal row.

GANGLION

Characteristics	Signs and Symptoms	Special Tests	Intervention
• Soft, round, and movable cyst filled with mucin • Common on the dorsal aspect of the wrist by the capsule or the tendon • May be caused by repetitive trauma	• "Bump" on the dorsal wrist area • Does not usually change in appearance with wrist position • Not usually painful • Can rupture on its own or with direct trauma	• Appearance	• Can be aspirated if symptomatic • Usually no PT, but if stiff after removal, paraffin and ROM exercises may help

OSTEOARTHRITIS

Characteristics	Signs and Symptoms	Special Tests	Intervention
• Uncommon at the wrist • Common at the thumb • Can occur from microtrauma or unknown etiology	• Morning stiffness • Heberden's nodes at DIP joints • Hypo- or hypermobility • Weakness • Pain	• X-ray • Positive grind test • Positive valgus/varus tests	• Splinting • Pain-free ROM • Pain modalities if acute • Paraffin • Mobilizations • Strengthening (isometrics) • Steroid shots • Trapeziectomy

RHEUMATOID ARTHRITIS (RA)

Characteristics	Signs and Symptoms	Special Tests	Intervention
• Chronic, systemic inflammatory disorder affecting synovial joints, especially the hand • 75% of patients with RA have wrist problems	• Increased local temperature, Bouchard's nodes, atrophy, stiffness, and swelling • Ulnar head syndrome (deformity in UD) • IP joint contractures • Can progress to dislocations	• Observation • X-ray • Lab tests	• PRICE if acute • Maintain alignment, mobility, and strength • Splints • Joint protection • Adaptive equipment • Medication • Surgery: joint reconstruction if severe

TENDON INJURIES

Characteristics	Signs and Symptoms	Special Tests	Intervention
• Can be on extensor or flexor tendons • Can be partial or complete tears, stretch or compressed injuries • Tendons within a sheath heal slower due to swelling impairing blood flow • Extensor injuries usually do not retract and are easier to manage • Common tears: flexor digitorum profundus (FDP [jersey finger]), extensor tendon (mallet finger) • Common tendinitis includes the FCU due usually to repetitive trauma	• Impaired motion and function • Pain • Swelling • Difficulty with contractions • May result in a stiff hand	• Medical exam • Positive sweater sign for ruptured FDP	• Almost always needs surgery • Treatment thereafter depends on MD and location and type of injury • Main goal: wound care, edema control, immobilization, and early controlled passive mobilization

——————— N O T E S ———————

CARPAL TUNNEL RELEASE

Characteristics	Signs and Symptoms	Special Tests	Intervention
• Open technique or endoscopic technique	• Both techniques entail a division of the flexor retinaculum to decompress the tunnel	• Surgical	• Immobilization in a volar splint for 2 weeks • AROM exercises for the fingers and thumb • After 1 week, edema control, ROM, scar massage if possible, and desensitization • Strengthening and functional exercises after 3 weeks

——— N O T E S ———

SPECIAL TESTS

FINKELSTEIN'S TEST

Purpose	Positive Test	Interpretation	Comments
• To see if there is tenosynovitis of the APL and the EPB	• Pain in these tendons when the wrist is ulnarly deviated	• Diagnostic for De Quervain's tenosynovitis, which indicates stenosis and inflammation	• Can cause slight pain in asymptomatic people if performed with the thumb tucked in a fist, which is not the original description of the test

MURPHY'S SIGN

Purpose	Positive Test	Interpretation	Comments
• To determine whether the lunate is dislocated	• The third metacarpal is level with the other metacarpal upon making a fist	• Indicates the lunate is dislocated	• The test is usually painless

JERSEY FINGER TEST

Purpose	Positive Test	Interpretation	Comments
• To determine if there is a tear in the FDP tendon	• There is no flexion at the distal phalanx on the affected finger while making a fist	• There is a rupture of the tendon	• Usually occurs in the middle finger • Also called sweater finger

GAMEKEEPER'S THUMB (VALGUS STRESS TEST)

Purpose	Positive Test	Interpretation	Comments
• To test for the integrity of the ulnar (medial) collateral ligament of the thumb	• Pain and/or laxity are present when an abduction force is applied to the thumb (MCP)	• Hypermobility or instability of the metacarpophalangeal joint	• The laxity may predispose to osteoarthritis • Also called skier's thumb

TINEL'S SIGN

Purpose	Positive Test	Interpretation	Comments
• To determine if there is neuritis of the median nerve • May be performed on other superficial nerves	• Tingling and/or pain ensue with tapping over the volar aspect of the wrist	• Indicates carpal tunnel syndrome	• Tingling means there is regeneration • Pain and tingling means there is injury and degeneration

PHALEN'S TEST

Purpose	Positive Test	Interpretation	Comments
• To see if there is median nerve compromise • 76% specific and 51% sensitive	• Paresthesias are felt as the patient maintains the wrist fully flexed for 1 minute	• Indicates carpal tunnel syndrome	• Can be done actively or passively, uni- or bilaterally

FROMENT'S SIGN

Purpose	Positive Test	Interpretation	Comments
• To see if there is paralysis of the adductor pollicis muscle • To test the function of the ulnar nerve	• There is flexion of the terminal phalanx of the thumb upon firmly grasping (key pinch) a piece of paper that is being pulled away	• Indicates ulnar nerve involvement • The flexor pollicis longus overpowers the extensors	• The adductor pollicis is innervated by the ulnar nerve

JEANNE'S SIGN

Purpose	Positive Test	Interpretation	Comments
• To assess the integrity of the ulnar nerve and hand function	• There is hyperextension of the metacarpophalangeal joint of the thumb during a key pinch	• Indicates ulnar entrapment	• Common with Froment's sign

GRIND TEST

Purpose	Positive Test	Interpretation	Comments
• To determine if there is arthrosis or synovitis	• Pain arises with compression of the thumb into the trapezium with rotation of the thumb	• Indicates joint pathology	• May be performed on other joints

FINGER EXTENSION TEST

Purpose	Positive Test	Interpretation	Comments
• To assess if there is dorsal wrist pathology • The test is valuable only to reproduce symptoms	• Pain is elicited when resistance to extension of the flexed wrist is applied to the extended fingers	• May indicate instability, synovitis, fracture, degeneration, or Kienböck's disease	• Not a very diagnostic test, as it only indicates there may be pathology, but does not distinguish type or location

FUNCTIONAL TESTS

Purpose	Positive Test	Interpretation	Comments
• To assess function (fine motor skills, dexterity)	• Can be measured against time and/or quality of motion	• Determines the patient's functional limitations	• Purdue pegboard, Baltimore therapeutic equipment (BTE), Moberg pick-up test, etc

———— N O T E S ————

CHAPTER FOUR

TEMPOROMANDIBULAR JOINT DISORDERS AND SURGERIES

ANTERIOR DISC DISPLACEMENT WITH REDUCTION

Characteristics	Signs and Symptoms	Special Tests	Intervention
• Most common temporo-mandibular joint (TMJ) dysfunction • The disc is anterior and medial to the condyle upon closing the mouth; during opening, the disc reduces/relocates • May be associated with cervical dysfunction, stress, myofascial pain syndrome, poor posture, and headaches • More common in females	• Reciprocal clicking with opening and closing • Jaw deviates to the side of the lesion • Slight decrease in lateral excursion to the opposite side • Increased pain with bruxism	• Based on signs	• Mobilization if hypomobile • Repositioning splint • Patient education in behavior modification: avoid nail biting, clenching, and wide mouth opening; start soft diet; proper posture • Isometrics • Muscle re-education/proprioception in opening without deviating • Massage/US • Biofeedback • Relaxation exercises • Address cervical component

─────── N O T E S ───────

ANTERIOR DISC DISPLACEMENT WITHOUT REDUCTION

Characteristics	Signs and Symptoms	Special Tests	Intervention
• The disc stays anteriorly displaced during all mandibular motions • There is less clicking as the disc is not reducing, but with more muscle guarding • Can lead to disc perforation and osteoarthritis if chronic	• Deflection to the same side of the dislocation • Decreased protrusion and lateral excursion to the opposite side • Jaw locked closed • If acute, there is decreased opening • If chronic, there is crepitus and more normal ROM	• Based on signs	• See previous table • Focus on mobilizations • May also use modalities as needed • Treatment is geared toward recapturing the disc • Surgery

CAPSULAR FIBROSIS

Characteristics	Signs and Symptoms	Special Tests	Intervention
• Capsular tightness, usually due to trauma, surgery, prolonged immobilization, or chronic capsulitis • May be associated with bruxism	• Decreased ROM in all planes if bilateral • TMJ pain, uni- or bilaterally • Deflection to the involved side if unilateral • Decreased lateral excursion to opposite side	• Based on signs • Differentiate between anterior disc displacement without reduction with a good history	• Mobilization • US • ROM exercises • Tongue blades to stretch • Self-mobilization • Soft tissue mobilization (STM)

CAPSULITIS AND SYNOVITIS

Characteristics	Signs and Symptoms	Special Tests	Intervention
• Inflammatory response of the TMJ • Usually due to trauma or post-surgically • Usually seen with disc dislocations • Associated with bruxism	• Preauricular pain • Usually no clicking • Decreased opening with capsulitis • Tender to palpate; with capsulitis, tenderness is on the lateral pole and with synovitis, on external auditory meatus	• Based on signs and symptoms	• Ice if acute • Heat if chronic • Phonophoresis • Mobilization • ROM exercises • Soft diet • Patient education • STM

TMJ SUBLUXATION

Characteristics	Signs and Symptoms	Special Tests	Intervention
• The condyle translates onto the articular tubercle then back to the articular eminence • Usually unilateral • Can cause synovitis	• There is usually clicking at the beginning of opening with hypermobility • If unilateral, the jaw deflects to the opposite side at the end of opening	• Based on signs • May hear/feel a "thud" • Increased joint space with palpation • Muscle imbalance	• Isometric exercises on the involved side • Proprioceptive exercises • Avoid excessive motion and aggravators • Patient education

TMJ DISLOCATION

Characteristics	Signs and Symptoms	Special Tests	Intervention
• One or both condyles are displaced forward onto the infratemporal fossa • Due to hypermobility or trauma	• The jaw deflects to the opposite side if unilateral • Jaw is locked open • May or may not be painful	• Based on signs	• Closed reduction • Strengthening exercises • Avoid wide opening of mouth • Proprioceptive exercises

OSTEOARTHRITIS

Characteristics	Signs and Symptoms	Special Tests	Intervention
• Insidious onset • Initially asymptomatic	• Crepitus and clicking • Deviation to the involved side at the end of opening and with protrusion • Morning stiffness/pain • Headaches, limited ROM, dizziness, and hearing problems	• Based on signs and symptoms	• Mobilization • Heat • ROM exercises as tolerated • Patient education • Postural exercises • Surgery

COMMON TMJ SURGERIES

Characteristics	Signs and Symptoms	Special Tests	Intervention
• Lysis and lavage • Discectomy • Discectomy with implant • Temporalis fascial graft • Costochondral graft • Total joint replacement • Can be done arthroscopically or via opened procedure	• Postsurgical inflammation • Decreased ROM • Pain	• Surgical	• Acute: ES, ice, AROM, liquid diet, controlled condylar rotation without translation, isometrics • Chronic: as above plus mobilizations without overpressure and progression to soft diet

——————— N O T E S ———————

CHAPTER FIVE

CERVICAL DISORDERS
AND
SPECIAL TESTS

CERVICAL STRAIN

Characteristics	Signs and Symptoms	Special Tests	Intervention
• Injury to a muscle due to excessive stretching or trauma, acceleration injury in a car accident (whiplash), or muscle imbalance • Ligaments may be affected if traumatic • May be associated with headaches	• Local, diffuse, and/or referred muscle pain • Tenderness and tightness • Muscle fatigue and burning • May have spasm and decreased ROM • Rest relieves it but causes stiffness	• Neurologic signs are negative • History • Behavior of symptoms • X-ray may show decreased lordosis • Test for alar ligament stability and for vertebral artery integrity	• Acute: rest, ice, ES, gentle AROM as tolerated • Medication • Subacute: heat, gentle stretching, postural education • Occipito-atlantal (O-A) releases • No mechanical traction is needed

——————— N O T E S ———————

POSTURAL SYNDROME

Characteristics	Signs and Symptoms	Special Tests	Intervention
• More common in women than in men 3:1 usually up to the age of 45 • Gradual onset usually due to poor sitting habits resulting in muscle overuse (excessive forward head) • Chronic • Poor posture • Worse at the end of the day and with stress; better with rest	• Faulty posture (forward head, rounded shoulder, kyphosis) • Hypomobility • Agonist weakness • Headaches • May have TMJ pain • Muscle fatigue and burning, especially upper trapezius • Pain on the head, neck, upper trapezius, and interscapular muscles with prolonged positions	• Postural exam shows faulty alignment • No history of trauma • Neurologic signs are negative • May have trigger points	• Stretching short anterior muscles • Strengthening weak posterior muscles • Patient education • Postural correction • Ergonomic assessment • Massage/heat • Stress management

—————— N O T E S ——————

RHEUMATOID ARTHRITIS

Characteristics	Signs and Symptoms	Special Tests	Intervention
• Chronic, systemic inflammatory disease with proliferation of synovial lining, cartilage destruction, and joint margin erosion • Can lead to instability due to transverse ligament and dens involvement • Occurs usually in the upper cervical area: C1 to C2	• Pain • Instability • Neurologic symptoms if more severe • Morning stiffness lasting at least 1 hour • Decreased ROM • May develop cervical myelopathy • Present in other joints usually bilaterally	• Alar ligament tests may be positive • Crepitus • Blood work positive for RA factor • X-rays • Elsewhere, nodules over bony prominences	• Medication • Cervical collar • Stabilization • Cold if flared up • Heat if stiff • Isometrics • No mobilizations or traction • Surgery if unstable

———— N O T E S ————

CERVICAL SPONDYLOSIS OR ARTHROSIS (DJD, DDD, OA)

Characteristics	Signs and Symptoms	Special Tests	Intervention
• Segmental degenerative disease common in adults and usually progressive • May cause osteophytes and hypomobility if degenerative • Can be due to hyper- or hypomobility • Joint space narrowing • May be due to previous injuries and/or wear and tear or normal aging • Common at C5, C6, and C7 • Can lead to stenosis or myelopathy	• Diffuse pain that eases with light activity • Aggravated with increased activity • Rest causes pain and stiffness • If facet is involved, it is usually worse with extension • If disc is involved, it is worse with flexion • Morning stiffness of less than 30 minutes • There may be crepitus • Tenderness to palpation	• Neurologic signs are negative unless there is nerve root involvement • Can be uni- or bilateral and refer symptoms up and down, related to neck position • May have intermittent pain • Decreased ROM if hypomobile • Shoulder girdle weakness	• Medication • Heat • AROM and gentle stretching • Submaximal isometrics if tolerated • Patient education and postural exercises • Cervical (cx) traction if no contraindications • Mobilizations if no RA or cord problems

Note: Also known as osteoarthritis (OA), degenerative joint disease (DJD), and degenerative disc disease (DDD).

THORACIC OUTLET SYNDROME (TOS)

Characteristics	Signs and Symptoms	Special Tests	Intervention
• Pressure on the neurovascular bundle in the supraclavicular fossa or costo-clavicular space • Females affected more than males (3:1) • Common in 30- to 40-year-olds • Easily confused with RSD, Raynaud's disease, herniated nucleus pulposus (HNP), myocardial infarction (MI), carcinoma, carpal tunnel syndrome, and ulnar neuropathy • Common due to poor prolonged postures or trauma • Can be due to elevated or hypomobile first rib, short pectoralis, and/or scalene muscles	• Local and/or distal disturbance of nerve and/or vascular function • Intense, constant, dull, throbbing pain, working or with the arm elevated during sleep • Can refer distally • All motions can cause pain • Swelling, numbness, and tingling (last two fingers) • Weakness in severe cases, especially on the hand intrinsics (C8-T1) • Decreased sensation on forearm and hand • Cyanosis of fingers, pallor, coldness • Subclavian bruit	• Adson's, Allen's, Halstead, and Roos tests may be positive • Pain with supraclavicular pressure • Doppler • Arteriogram • EMG/NCV • Observation • Trigger points • Differentiation with ulnar neuropathy: TOS may have sensory deficit on ulnar aspect of the limb and motor involvement of thenar muscles	• Decrease precipitating factors • Medication • Postural education • Heat • Traction • ROM exercises • Scalene and pectoralis minor stretches • First rib mobilizations • Arm sling • Cervical collar • Transcutaneous electrical nerve stimulation (TENS) • Strengthening • Surgery (first rib resection)

MYOFASCIAL PAIN SYNDROME

Characteristics	Signs and Symptoms	Special Tests	Intervention
• Differs from fibromyalgia in that trigger points and symptoms are regional • Common in scapular area, but can occur elsewhere • Often recurs • More common in women older than 30 • Usually gradual onset • Can be associated with poor posture	• Regional pain • Referred pain and/or paresthesias in a predictable pattern when pressure is applied to active trigger points • Upper back weakness • Headaches • Decreased cervical ROM usually due to muscle tightness	• Positive twitch response • Local active trigger points • Tissue texture abnormalities • Differentiate from fibromyalgia: diffuse soft tissue pain, sleep disturbance, fatigue, and at least 11 out of 18 tender points	• ES with US • Trigger point pressure/massage • Stretching • Strengthening • Aerobics • Postural correction • Patient education • Spray and stretch • Trigger point injections

─────── N O T E S ───────

FACET IMPINGEMENT

Characteristics	Signs and Symptoms	Special Tests	Intervention
• Also known as facet locking, subluxation, wry neck, and acute torticollis • Acute painful facet joint disorder • Usually due to sudden, unguarded movement with little or no trauma • Can last 1 to 2 weeks • Meniscoid inclusions block motion • Congenital torticollis is sternoclediomastoid (SCM) contracture with sidebending (SB) to the same side and rotation (ROT) to the opposite side, common during delivery, treated with stretching	• Spasms and guarding, especially SCM • Usually locked neck: SB and ROT to same side (protective posture); can lock in forward flexion or backward bending (FF or BB) • Better with rest • Worse if trying to straighten out • No increased pain with motion to affected side • Tenderness over the facet • Can be very painful • Usually unilateral at C3 to C5	• True neurologic signs are usually negative • Pain can be felt in sensory distribution of spinal nerve root • Sharp pain with protective deformity • SB and ROT away from affected side can increase the symptoms (a facet sprain is similar but is usually due to trauma)	• Manual traction in line with the deformity, gradually working to the painful direction • PROM away from the pain • Mobilizations on hypomobile joints • Heat or cold • Cervical isometrics for stabilization

ACUTE DISC HERNIATION

Characteristics	Signs and Symptoms	Special Tests	Intervention
• HNP usually posteriorly • More common at C5, C6, and C7 unilateral and posterolateral • Usually due to trauma, like heavy lifting or sudden exertion • Can occur due to degenerative changes if the onset is slow • Common in patients with forward head posture	• Similar pain to facet impingement • If small, it may ease with BB and SB to the opposite direction • Worse with overpressure and motion to the same side • Neck pain and paresthesias can radiate to fingers and/or the scapular region (Cloward's areas)	• Positive neuro signs • Worse with sneezing and coughing • Numbness and tingling • Altered deep tendon reflexes (DTRs) and sensation • Late atrophy and weakness • Positive compression, distraction, and Spurling tests • Bakody sign may be positive if C5 to C6 is involved	• Cold • Traction • Extension usually helps • Positioning • Patient education • Postural exercises • Soft collar in acute stages • Gentle stretching • Progress to stabilization • Surgery in about 20% of cases

———— N O T E S ————

CERVICAL RADICULOPATHY

Characteristics	Signs and Symptoms	Special Tests	Intervention
• Due to compression, irritation, and/or stretching of the nerve root • May also be due to lateral spinal stenosis • Common in women older than 35 • Common at C5 to C7 • Can come with HNP, facet DJD, spasm, and/or decreased intervertebral foraminal (IVF) space • Frequently unilateral with poor posture • Compression may cause neuropraxia or axonotmesis • Nerve root lesions have true neurologic signs	• UE radicular symptoms • Deep burning pain • Aggravated with movements that close the intervertebral foramen • Referred pain • Decreased or absent DTRs • Numbness, burning • Decreased sensation on defined dermatomes • Weakness, especially with repetitive activities • Atrophy as it progresses • Headaches	• If C7-8 is involved, the symptoms can decrease by holding the forearm • If C4 to C6 is involved, patients may rest the arm over the head (Bakody sign) • May have positive compression, distraction, and Spurling tests • Imaging, EMG, NCV	• Medication • Traction if there are no contraindications • Rest/collar • Ice progressing to heat • Postural correction • Positioning • AROM • Soft tissue mobilization • Patient education • ES and strengthening • Surgery if severe

Note: Also known as nerve root compression or cervicobrachialgia.

CERVICAL SPINAL STENOSIS

Characteristics	Signs and Symptoms	Special Tests	Intervention
• Narrowing of the spinal and/or intervertebral canal • Associated with DJD (acquired) • May be due to ossification of the posterior longitudinal ligament or hypertrophic facets • Can cause nerve root and cord compression (myelopathy) • More common in men (2:1) older than 50 • Can also be congenital • Commonly seen in football players	• Pain may decrease with flexion • Worse with extension • Numbness and tingling uni- or bilaterally • Altered reflexes • Weakness, especially with prolonged tasks • Distal atrophy	• Imaging • Cluster of signs and symptoms	• Heat • Cervical flexion • Patient education • Positioning • Traction • Refer to MD if severe neurologic signs are present • Surgery

SPRENGEL'S DEFORMITY

Characteristics	Signs and Symptoms	Special Tests	Intervention
• Congenital, undescended scapula and hypoplastic muscles often associated with Klippel-Feil syndrome	• Decreased muscle strength, especially scapular abductors • Decreased ROM	• Neurologic signs • Webbing or shortening of the neck	• Surgical for cosmetic reasons and to increase ROM

BRACHIAL PLEXUS INJURIES

Characteristics	Signs and Symptoms	Special Tests	Intervention
• May be due to stretch trauma • If during infancy, it is called Erb's palsy (C5 to C6), Klumpke's palsy (C8-T1), or combination of both (obstetric problems: breech or complicated cephalic birth, but can be traumatic, neoplastic, infectious, surgical, etc) • Also called "backpack paralysis" in sports, due to compressive force from the straps on the clavicle or first rib (TOS symptoms)	• Absent DTRs • UE paralysis with arm held in IR and adduction without elbow flexion • Atrophy • Altered sensation and limited activities of daily living (ADLs) • If backpack injury: weakness, especially on axillary and radial nerves, rarely painful with minor sensation changes • Temperature and color alterations may be present due to autonomic nervous system (ANS) damage	• Refer to signs and symptoms • EMG to localize extent of lesion • NCV to localize level of lesion • Increase symptoms with SB and ROT away from symptoms	• ES for muscle reeducation • Strengthening • Splinting UE • Microsurgery for nerve grafting and repair • Backpack injuries are usually nonoperative, where recovery usually occurs after elimination of compression forces but can take several years

N O T E S

BRACHIAL NEURITIS

Characteristics	Signs and Symptoms	Special Tests	Intervention
• Acute onset of shoulder pain that can be bilateral • Unknown but possibly due to trauma or infection • Incidence 1:100,000 • Affects all ages, especially men between 30 and 70 • 90% of patients recover in 3 years	• Shoulder pain radiating to neck and UEs • Weakness develops as pain subsides and progresses to atrophy • Usually confused with other shoulder pathology due to similarity of symptoms	• EMG • MRI • Involvement of muscles not inervated by the brachial plexus • Must differentiate with rotator cuff lesions, impingement syndrome, capsulitis, and radiculopathy	• Rest • Analgesics • ROM exercises as pain decreases • Strengthening and scapular stabilization

CERVICAL MYELOPATHY

Characteristics	Signs and Symptoms	Special Tests	Intervention
• Spinal cord compression usually due to spurs, HNP, or thickened ligamentum flavum • Common in people older than 55, usually due to spondylosis • Cord compression can occur with or without motion, especially flexion and extension	• Neck pain in one-third of patients • Unusual hand sensations • Weakness, spasticity, incoordination, gait disturbance, decreased sensation, increased DTRs, clonus, Babinski • Incontinence in latter stages	• MRI, computed tomography (CT) scan, and plain films • Signs and symptoms	• Refer to MD if acute

STINGERS

Characteristics	Signs and Symptoms	Special Tests	Intervention
• Also known as "burners," cervical nerve impingement or upper brachial plexus injuries, seen mostly in football players • Occurs with downward or backward blow to the shoulder with cervical SB away from side of the blow • Incidence increases if there is congenital cervical stenosis	• Burning from supraclavicular area to the hand with numbness and tingling, not dermatomal • Usually resolves in 1 to 2 minutes and has no true neck pain • Weakness can develop later in the deltoids and rotator cuff muscles	• Based on signs, symptoms, and mechanism of injury	• Allow symptoms to subside. If no weakness, athlete can return to sports. If symptoms persist, then no sports • Strengthen neck/shoulder muscles; cervical roll to prevent SB

KLIPPEL-FEIL SYNDROME

Characteristics	Signs and Symptoms	Special Tests	Intervention
• Congenital fusion of the C-spine that can result in altered central nervous system (CNS) • Short neck, low hairline, decreased ROM and hearing	• Seen in infants and children, mostly girls • May have headaches, neck pain, and weakness	• Observation • X-rays	• Maintain ROM and strength • Pain modalities • Brace • Surgery

SPECIAL TESTS

COMPRESSION TEST

Purpose	Positive Test	Interpretation	Comments
• To reproduce pain and/or paresthesias due to cervical nerve compression	• Symptoms appear with downward pressure on the head with the patient in sitting or supine position	• Radicular pain indicates nerve root irritation, and radiculopathy indicates compression (the intervertebral foramen closes)	• May incorporate cervical rotation to the compression

DISTRACTION TEST

Purpose	Positive Test	Interpretation	Comments
• To decrease the above symptoms	• Radiculopathy and/or radicular or cervical pain diminish when the neck is distracted while the patient is supine	• Nerve root compression is relieved due to widening of the foramen	• If the test is positive, traction should be a component of therapy

——————— N O T E S ———————

SPURLING TEST

Purpose	Positive Test	Interpretation	Comments
• To reproduce radicular pain and/or paresthesias due to foraminal compression	• Symptoms appear with cervical sidebending and extension followed by vertical compression with the patient sitting	• Nerve root compression on the side of the sidebending • May be indicative of disc herniation, spurs, or facet involvement	• If symptoms appear without compression, there is no need to include the compression • Use caution • Test first for vertebral artery

BAKODY SIGN

Purpose	Positive Test	Interpretation	Comments
• To determine if there is cervical nerve root compression	• Radicular pain decreases when the patient rests the affected arm on his or her head	• Indicates nerve root compression at C5 to C6, usually due to an HNP • Usually the patient adopts this antalgic position automatically	• By elevating the suprascapular nerve, the traction of the lower trunk of the brachial plexus decreases • Also called shoulder abduction test

——————— N O T E S ———————

DIZZINESS TEST

Purpose	Positive Test	Interpretation	Comments
• To determine if this symptom lies in the vestibular system or vertebral artery	• The patient rotates the neck then the shoulders (upper body) fully to both sides. If dizziness occurs with both motions, the problem is arterial	• The vertebral arteries become "kinked" with rotation from above or from below	• Body motion without head motion should not cause vertigo or dizziness

UPPER LIMB TENSION TESTS

Purpose	Positive Test	Interpretation	Comments
• To reproduce the patient's UE symptoms by stressing neural tissue • There are four different positions or "biases" for different nerves • Does not seem to be a very sensitive test, as some individuals have a positive test and are asymptomatic	• ULTT 1, which is most common, identifies median nerve root (C5 to C7): slowly depress the shoulder while supine, bring arm into abduction, extension, and supination with wrist and fingers extended. If positive, the symptoms are sharp pain, burning, paresthesias, and/or tingling (dermatomal)	• Indicates nerve irritation, usually at the nerve root	• Different positions stress different nerves • Also stresses other tissues • Test the uninvolved side first • If symptoms appear early during the test, do not proceed • May test distal to proximal or vice versa

VERTEBRAL ARTERY TEST

Purpose	Positive Test	Interpretation	Comments
• To determine if there is vascular insufficiency	• With the patient sitting, he or she actively rotates and extends the head. A positive test results in vertigo, nausea, nystagmus, syncope, or blurred vision	• Indicates arterial compromise due to spurs, atherosclerosis, facet subluxation • Differentiate with vestibular dysfunction where Rhomberg and unilateral stance may be positive	• Cervical rotation causes arterial compression usually on the ipsilateral side. If positive, avoid rotation • Can be done passively in supine • Also called Barre-Lieou sign

ALAR TEST

Purpose	Positive Test	Interpretation	Comments
• To determine the integrity of the alar ligament • Subluxation of the atlas on the axis can be observed and palpated: a prominent C2 spinous process is noted with cervical flexion	• Palpate C2 in supine and slightly side-bend the neck while flexed. A positive test shows C2 did not move immediately as it should	• Indicates dens fracture, ligament tear, instability • More common in patients with RA	• Should be performed on patients with history of trauma. Refer to MD if transoral x-rays have not been done and there is history of trauma

ALLEN'S TEST

Purpose	Positive Test	Interpretation	Comments
• To determine if there is TOS	• If the test is positive, the patient's pulse decreases when the arm is in the throwing position and the neck turned the other way	• Indicates neurovascular compression of the subclavian artery and brachial plexus that may be due to cervical rib, abnormal scalenes, poor posture, trauma, or arteriosclerosis	• May show false positives • The test is more valid if it is positive only on the symptomatic side

ADSON'S TEST

Purpose	Positive Test	Interpretation	Comments
• To determine if there is TOS	• If the test is positive, the patient's pulse decreases with the extended neck rotated to the same side of the extended and abducted arm, while holding his or her breath	• Same as above • All TOS tests are more valid if they reproduce the symptoms • Need two or more tests to be positive to assist with the diagnosis	• May show false positives • If negative, patient should turn head to the opposite side • The test is more valid if positive only on the affected side

ROOS TEST

Purpose	Positive Test	Interpretation	Comments
• To determine if there is TOS	• With the arms in the "hands up" position, the patient opens and closes the hands for 3 minutes. The test is positive if there is numbness and tingling, pain, marked heaviness, and/or inability to keep the arms up	• Indicates TOS and vascular insufficiency	• Minor complaints of fatigue are normal • May also be done quickly for 15 repetitions • Also known as "hands up" test

HALSTEAD MANEUVER

Purpose	Positive Test	Interpretation	Comments
• To determine if there is TOS	• Apply a downward traction to the affected UE while feeling the patient's pulse as he or she extends and rotates the neck to the opposite side	• Indicates TOS if the pulse decreases or disappears	• Same as other TOS tests

LHERMITTE'S SIGN

Purpose	Positive Test	Interpretation	Comments
• To identify cervical myelopathy	• When sitting, the patient flexes the neck, and if the test is positive, he or she will have sharp pain down the spine and into the extremities	• Indicates dural irritation from cervical cord compression	• May be present in patients with multiple sclerosis • Notify/refer to MD

CERVICAL NONORGANIC SIGNS

Purpose	Positive Test	Interpretation	Comments
• To identify patients with abnormal illness behavior	• Sensory disturbance nondermatomal • Motor disturbance non-myotomal • Overreaction (rubbing, clutching the area, and sighing)	• Only one positive sign should be discounted	• The patient may also have increased tenderness to light touch and decreased cervical rotation

NOTES

CHAPTER SIX

THORACIC DISORDERS

FACET HYPOMOBILITY SYNDROME

Characteristics	Signs and Symptoms	Special Tests	Intervention
• Restricted joint motion usually due to trauma, degenerative changes, or poor posture	• Localized pain with motion and sometimes with inhalation • Normal kyphosis is altered (increase or decrease) • Tenderness • Positional faults • Decreased segmental mobility • May have decreased ROM	• Positive passive intervertebral motion testing (PIVM) • Positive spring test	• Heat • Joint mobilization • Postural education • Stretching and strengthening • Breathing exercises

FACET HYPERMOBILITY SYNDROME

Characteristics	Signs and Symptoms	Special Tests	Intervention
• Increased mobility usually due to trauma (pushing, pulling, and/or reaching) or from muscle imbalances or compensations above or below a restricted segment • Can occur from excessive joint "popping"	• Pain usually after increased activity (fatigue) • Increased muscle tone • Tenderness on associated ligaments • Positional faults • Increased segmental mobility • Clicking; need to "pop"	• Positive PIVM • Positive spring test	• Restore neighboring hypomobility • Strengthening • Postural education • Bracing if more involved • Stabilization exercises

POSTURAL SYNDROMES

Characteristics	Signs and Symptoms	Special Tests	Intervention
• Dowager's hump: upper T-spine kyphosis seen in osteoporotic and/or post-menopausal women • Kyphosis and scoliosis: spinal curve alterations, usually nonpainful if mild	• Dowager's hump: hypomobility in upper T-spine with a hump and mild tenderness • Curve alterations may have hypo- and hypermobility • Postural deficits may be visible	• Observation • X-ray	• Postural, stretching, and strengthening exercises • Patient education • Bracing • Surgery for scoliosis if severe

Notes: Dowager's hump, scoliosis, kyphosis, and hyperlordosis are types of postural syndromes.

THORACIC HNP

Characteristics	Signs and Symptoms	Special Tests	Intervention
• Very rare • More frequent in men older than 50 at T11 and 12 • Usually due to axial compression • Can cause cord compression	• May have radicular pain • Pain is usually constant, dull, and burning • Increased kyphosis • Pain with breathing	• Imaging	• Modalities • Bracing • Rest • Postural exercises • Extension and stabilization exercises

T4 Syndrome

Characteristics	Signs and Symptoms	Special Tests	Intervention
• Associated with hypomobility at T4 but can occur at other levels • ANS may be involved • Predisposing factors include trauma (motor vehicle accident [MVA]) or unaccustomed activities • Not very common	• Pain and paresthesias down the arm that does not follow a dermatomal distribution, with the hand always involved • Tenderness • Head and neck pain • Hyper- or hypomobility	• Positive ULTT • Positive slump test in some patients	• Mobilizations • Postural correction • Gentle neural stretching • Strengthening as symptoms decrease • Traction and modalities for pain may help

Compression Fractures

Characteristics	Signs and Symptoms	Special Tests	Intervention
• Due to minor trauma in the elderly, usually from osteoporosis • More common in women older than 60 • Common at T11-12, L1-2 • May occur spontaneously	• Acute pain after trauma, especially with motion • Very limited extension and rotation	• X-ray	• Acute: bed rest and pain modalities • Walking program after • Extension/stabilization exercises if tolerated • Bracing • Patient education • Vertebroplasty (percutaneous or balloon augmented) to restore the vertebral height

SCHEUERMANN'S DISEASE (JUVENILE KYPHOSIS)

Characteristics	Signs and Symptoms	Special Tests	Intervention
• Disorder of the epiphyseal growth plate of the vertebral body • Results in anterior wedging of the vertebra • Etiology is unknown but is associated with increased activity and poor posture • Common in 12- to 18-year-old boys • Common at T9 and may involve five vertebra • Can lead to DDD, cord compression, spondylolysis, and stenosis	• Mild, localized pain • Kyphosis • Hypomobility	• X-ray shows Schmörl's nodes (HNP in vertebral body), wedging, and narrow intervertebral space • Decreased bone mineral density	• Postural exercises, especially in extension • Stretching, especially hamstrings and pectoralis • Strengthening scapular adductors and paraspinals • Bracing • Biofeedback

N O T E S

COSTOCHONDRITIS

Characteristics	Signs and Symptoms	Special Tests	Intervention
• Also known as Tietze's syndrome or costochondrosis • Irritation of costochondral junction • Can be due to trauma, infection, surgical complication, arthritis, bronchitis, or unknown • Common at fourth rib and in teens, L > R	• Localized anterior chest wall pain, especially with palpation and after a persistent cough • Pain may radiate to the shoulder and arm	• Palpation and history • Imaging	• Iontophoresis • Phonophoresis • Mobilizations • Medication • Surgical resection

—————— NOTES ——————

RIB DYSFUNCTION (HYPOMOBILITY)

Characteristics	Signs and Symptoms	Special Tests	Intervention
• Usually associated with costovertebral, costotransverse, and/or costochondral joint problems • Usually hypomobile but can be hypermobile • Can be due to trauma, DJD, ankylosis, or postural deficits • Common at T8 to T10 • Gradual or sudden onset	• Localized pain anywhere along the rib and its attachments • Pain may refer laterally and be felt with breathing and sneezing • Tenderness • Altered rib position • Restricted motion: inhalation (rib does not move up) or exhalation (rib does not move down) restriction	• Palpation • Positive spring test • Hypomobility	• Mobilization, first of posterior joints • Intercostal muscle stretching • Breathing exercises • Muscle energy techniques • Postural exercises

— N O T E S —

Diffuse Idiopathic Skeletal Hyperostosis (dish)*

Characteristics	Signs and Symptoms	Special Tests	Intervention
• Calcification of ligaments, especially the anterior longitudinal ligament (not only in the thoracic spine) • Spurs fuse forming bony bridges • Affects more men (2:1) older than 65 than women • Etiology is unknown; possible link to diabetes • Incidence is 5% to 10% of the population • Can present in peripheral joints (knee, elbow, heel [enthesopathy])	• Decreased mobility • Decreased lordosis in the lumbar spine • Dysphagia from the cervical spine due to spurs • Can cause stenosis • Can cause paraplegia and fractures in severe cases • Aches, stiffness, and radicular pain • Mostly asymmetrical • Worsens with use or prolonged rest	• X-ray: bony bridging in at least four vertebrae (anterolateral aspect) without disc degeneration • Differential diagnosis with ankylosing spondylitis: none to minimal sacroiliac joint (SIJ) involvement, no osteoporosis or abnormal disc space, and no inflammation	• Heat • Maintain AROM without forcing motion • Restore function • Pain modalities if severe • No traction • No mobilization if bridging is present • Surgery

Notes: Also known as Forestier's disease.

HERPES ZOSTER

Characteristics	Signs and Symptoms	Special Tests	Intervention
• Viral infection of the dorsal ganglion of one or more nerve roots, known as shingles • Women older than 70 are affected more than men • Believed to be due to dormant chicken pox reactivated by stress • Self-limiting, lasting 2 to 3 weeks • Seems more prevalent during the summer	• Severe pain resulting in postherpetic neuralgia in 50% of cases • Dermatomal distribution of pain and skin eruptions along rib cage, but may extend elsewhere (eg, face)	• Observation of dermatomal lesions • Severe complaints of pain	• Antiviral and pain medication • Pulsed US • Cold (no heat) • TENS

—————— N O T E S ——————

CHAPTER SEVEN

LUMBAR DISORDERS
AND
SPECIAL TESTS

LUMBAR SPRAIN

Characteristics	Signs and Symptoms	Special Tests	Intervention
• Frequent on iliolumbar ligament • Usually due to forced flexion with contralateral sidebending/rotation • Muscles may also be affected • Common in patients under 30	• Unilateral low back pain (LBP) on sacroiliac and lumbosacral regions • Pain with FF, BB, SB away, and rotation toward the affected side • May have muscle guarding • Decreased trunk ROM • No true neurologic signs, but may cause referred pain	• Palpation • Rule out other disorders • Muscle guarding	• Rest a few days; avoid stressing ligaments • Pain modalities • Progress to gentle stretching exercises • Stabilization • Patient education in body mechanics/lifting

MECHANICAL LOW BACK PAIN

Characteristics	Signs and Symptoms	Special Tests	Intervention
• Also known as postural syndrome • Due to mechanical deformation of soft tissue from prolonged static forces • Common in sedentary people younger than 30	• Local pain that is never constant • Movement does not alter the symptoms • No neurologic signs	• Postural exam • Patient history	• Postural correction • Patient education • Stretching, strengthening, and conditioning

FACET IMPINGEMENT OR SYNDROME (LUMBAGO, LOCKING)

Characteristics	Signs and Symptoms	Special Tests	Intervention
• Facet sprain leading to inflammation, spasm, and pain • Joint capsule is caught between articular surfaces • Frequently caused by flexion/rotation injury but may also occur from extension/rotation • Onset of pain is immediate	• Pain decreases with flexion and increases with extension or SB to same side (joint compression), especially at end ranges • No true neurologic signs, but pain may refer to buttock and thigh • Difficulty straightening up • Relieved with rest • May have a positional fault and muscle guarding • Hypomobility/ decreased ROM	• History (mechanism of injury) • Forward flexed posture • Positional fault	• Joint rest and pain modalities • AROM when tolerated, gradually working out of the locked position • PROM: traction and rotation to gap the joint • Mobilization • Patient education • Traction • Stabilization if the segment is unstable

LUMBAR SPONDYLOSIS (DDD, DJD, OA)

Characteristics	Signs and Symptoms	Special Tests	Intervention
• Segmental degenerative disease • Spurs are present, leading to hypomobility • Joint space narrowing • More common at L4-L5, S1	• Pain eases with motion • Increases with prolonged positions • Does not radiate unless severe (stenosis) • Local LBP • Morning stiffness	• X-ray: decreased disc space, narrow intervertebral foramen, and osteophytes	• Heat • Flexion and extension exercises • Mobilization • Traction • Patient education • Conditioning

SPONDYLOLYSIS AND SPONDYLOLISTHESIS

Characteristics	Signs and Symptoms	Special Tests	Intervention
• Spondylolysis: defect (stress/fatigue fracture) of pars interarticularis • Spondylolisthesis: vertebra above slips forward on the one below • Common at L5-S1 • Four grades • In young patients, it is usually traumatic (gymnasts 70%) or congenital • In the older population, it is usually degenerative • 10% incidence	• Asymptomatic if stable • If painful, it can be local or diffuse, uni- or bilateral • Symptoms can ease with trunk flexion and increase with extension • May have true neurologic signs and radicular pain • Hyperlordosis • May coexist with HNP • Hypermobility/instability	• X-ray ("Scottie dog") • May palpate a "step-off" • Positive stork extension test	• Flexion exercises • Stabilization • Bracing • Abdominal strengthening • Patient education • Avoid extension and mobilization of the involved segment • Surgery (fusion) if more severe/unstable

———— N O T E S ————

PIRIFORMIS SYNDROME

Characteristics	Signs and Symptoms	Special Tests	Intervention
• Entrapment of the sciatic nerve as it passes the sciatic notch under or through the muscle • More common in women (6:1) • May be due to trigger points, trauma, pressure, spasm, SIJ dysfunction	• Weight shifting while sitting • Sciatic symptoms • Tenderness on the muscle • May have SIJ pain • Pain usually sudden, deep, and aching • Tightness	• Piriformis palpation causes pain • Pain with resisted abduction and ER • EMG • Imaging • Need to differentiate with other sciatic problems	• US/massage • Piriformis stretching • Correct muscle imbalances • Decrease mechanical impingement • Address SIJ problems if present

——— N O T E S ———

ANKYLOSING SPONDYLITIS

Characteristics	Signs and Symptoms	Special Tests	Intervention
• Chronic and inflammatory rheumatic disease • Causes spinal fusion • More common in men than women (3:1) younger than 40 with gradual onset • Usually starts in the SIJ and progresses up the axial skeleton • Can be present at the hips, chest, ischial tuberosities, and greater trochanters • Enthesitis (inflammation at bone-tendon junction), especially at Achilles' tendon	• Morning stiffness >30 minutes • Pain is better with activity and worsens with chronicity • Buttock ache • Getting out of bed at night due to pain • Neurologic signs are only present if nerve roots are involved • Heel pain • Eye disorders • Sacroiliitis • All spinal ROMs are decreased • Decreased chest expansion • Rigid gait • Hip flexor contractures	• Blood test (increased erythrocyte sedimentation rate [ESR] and positive HLA-B27) • X-ray ("bamboo spine," "whiskering") • Age may help differentiate between AS and DISH	• Medication • Exercises, including breathing exercises • Decrease prolonged positions • Maintain ROM and strength • Stretching and functional exercises

——— N O T E S ———

RADICULOPATHY (NERVE ROOT COMPRESSION SYNDROME)

Characteristics	Signs and Symptoms	Special Tests	Intervention
• Impingement or irritation of spinal nerve root • Usually caused by HNP but also by tumors, DJD, stenosis, fractures, or congenital problems • Axonal conduction is blocked, hence numbness if on sensory nerve and weakness if on motor nerve • May or may not come with radicular pain that causes shooting and lancinating pain 2 inches wide down the lower extremity (LE), due to inflammation (HNP)	• True neurologic signs (weakness, reflex, and sensory changes) • Burning, deep pain specific to one nerve root • Nerve root adhesions (adverse mechanical neural tension) have same signs and symptoms but due to scar adhesions, usually postsurgically. Prevented and treated with straight leg raise (SLR) and slump stretching, avoiding irritability. Radiculitis is also similar but due to inflammation	• Positive SLR and other peripheral nerve provocation tests such as slump and prone knee bend tests • Imaging	• Long-axis distraction of the involved lower extremity if tolerated • Positioning • Traction • Muscular and neural stretching as tolerated • Temporary modalities • Extension exercises if due to posterior HNP • Medication • Surgery if severe

DISC DISORDERS

Characteristics	Signs and Symptoms	Special Tests	Intervention
• HNP: displacement of nucleus beyond normal confines of the annulus • Four degrees: 1. Intraspongy herniation from end-plate fracture (Schmörl's node) 2. Protrusion (no nuclear material escapes outer annulus) 3. Extrusion (nuclear material escapes into the spinal canal) 4. Sequestration (free fragment) • Also classified as contained or noncontained • Most common posterolaterally at L4-S1 • Usually due to cumulative effects	• Degree 1 is usually asymptomatic except for LBP with FF • Degree 2 causes LBP in 25- to 40-year-olds that can progress distally if nerve root is involved with positive neurologic signs, or referred pain from sinuvertebral nerve without these signs • Degrees 3 and 4 have above symptoms increased • May present with lateral shift and decreased lordosis • Decreased ROM • Decreased function • Increased pain with flexion (sitting, bending)	• Positive neurologic signs if nerve root is involved • Symptoms may increase with flexion, coughing, and sneezing • May have bowel, bladder, and sexual dysfunction • If the HNP is medial to the nerve root, there may be a list to the involved side, and, if lateral, the list is opposite • Imaging • May have positive peripheral nerve provocation tests	• Correct lateral shift and lumbar kyphosis • Centralize symptoms • Usually extension exercises for posterior lesions • Patient education • Positioning • Traction • Stabilization exercises • Surgery if unbearable or all measures have failed

SPINAL STENOSIS

Characteristics	Signs and Symptoms	Special Tests	Intervention
• Narrowing of the spinal and/or intervertebral canal • Can be due to DJD or may be congenital • Progressive and irreversible • Can cause root and cord compression, HNP, and spondylolisthesis • More common in men (2:1) older than 50 • History of long-standing LBP • More common in lower lumbar spine	• Pain lessens with flexion, sitting, and squatting • Worse walking, especially downhill, with activity or extension • Numbness and tingling uni- or bilaterally • May have bowel and bladder problems and saddle anesthesia • Decreased ankle jerk, especially after exercising • Weakness • Calf cramps and neurogenic claudication	• Imaging • Cluster of signs and symptoms • Lower extremity symptoms take longer to go away compared to vascular claudication • Bicycle test • Check pedal pulse to differentiate with vascular claudication	• Flexion • Patient education • Traction • Refer to MD if there are severe neurologic signs • Epidural steroid injections • Surgery (decompression)

COCCYGODYNIA

Characteristics	Signs and Symptoms	Special Tests	Intervention
• Painful condition of the coccyx • Usually due to direct trauma (falling on the buttocks)	• Painful sitting and straining • Tenderness • May have positional fault	• X-ray	• Direct mobilization • Ultrasound • Coccygeal pillow

CAUDA EQUINA SYNDROME

Characteristics	Signs and Symptoms	Special Tests	Intervention
• Usually due to trauma, neoplasm, or massive disc herniation • Bilateral polyradicular root syndrome • Can occur at any age • Medical emergency	• Pain can be acute or gradually increasing in lower back (LB) and legs • Saddle anesthesia • Loss of bowel and bladder control and sexual function	• Imaging • Positive SLR • Areflexia • Gastrocnemius weakness • Limited motion • Paresthesias	• Immediate surgery

NONORGANIC DISEASE

Characteristics	Signs and Symptoms	Special Tests	Intervention
• Psychogenic LBP • History is dramatic	• Symptoms hardly ease • Few objective signs • Inconsistency • Hypersensitivity • Cogwheel weakness	• Waddell's tests	• Aggressive strengthening and conditioning • Refer back to MD

Note: Other structural low back problems include facet tropism, lumbarization, and sacralization.

POST-LAMINECTOMY

Characteristics	Signs and Symptoms	Special Tests	Intervention
• Removal of bone between the base of the spinous process and facet • A bilateral laminectomy is removal of the spinous process and both laminae • Laminoplasty is enlargement of the spinal canal by excising the laminae and elevating the remaining bone tissue	• Indicated for large central protrusions or extrusions resulting in severe progressive neurological deficits and paresis/paralysis	• Surgical	• SLR stretching to avoid nerve root adhesions • Keep lordosis • Modalities and ambulation in acute phase • Progress to stabilization, strengthening, flexibility, and conditioning

POST-FUSION

Characteristics	Signs and Symptoms	Special Tests	Intervention
• Disc excision and removal of the end plates on both sides • The disc space is filled with bone graft • Also performed on the cervical spine	• Indicated for instability and spondylolisthesis • OK if spinal motion is limited	• Surgical	• Bracing until solid fusion • Progress to above exercises as indicated by MD • No traction for at least 1 year

SPECIAL TESTS

STRAIGHT LEG RAISE TEST (SLR)

Purpose	Positive Test	Interpretation	Comments
• To reproduce the patient's low back and/or leg symptoms • Symptoms indicate a problem at the level of the nerve root • Pain after 70 degrees may be from the lumbar spine or the SIJ • This and the next three tests are considered peripheral nerve provocation tests	• Passively lift the leg to pain or tension, lower it slightly, and dorsiflex the foot, and if this sensitizing maneuver does not reproduce the pain, then flex the neck (Lindner's sign). If symptoms are reproduced, the test is positive but not 100% diagnostic of a herniated disc	• Indicates nerve root compromise usually from a herniated disc (before 70 degrees) • The pain is due to stretching the sciatic nerve or its roots • Need to rule out hamstring tightness • Record the angle where symptoms were reproduced • The test is more diagnostic if positive below 30 degrees	• May combine with neck flexion, hip internal rotation, inversion, or eversion for further provocation • If pain arises on the opposite side (crossover sign), it is very diagnostic of a space-occupying lesion (large disc protrusion medial to the nerve root) • Also called Lasegue's test

——————— N O T E S ———————

PRONE KNEE BENDING

Purpose	Positive Test	Interpretation	Comments
• To reproduce the patient's lumbar, anterior thigh, or buttock/SI pain	• While prone, fully flex the knee passively while in a neutral position • May be modified to flex the knee toward the opposite buttock, or Yeoman's test is used when the hip is extended with the knee flexed	• Indicates L2 to L3 nerve root lesion if there is lumbar, SI, and/or anterior thigh pain without tightness. If there is tightness and no pain, there is a tight rectus femoris muscle • Culprit area can be implicated based on location of symptoms	• If the hip flexes during the test, it also indicates rectus femoris tightness • The femoral nerve stretches with this maneuver • Also called Ely's test or Nachlas test

KNEE FLEXION TEST

Purpose	Positive Test	Interpretation	Comments
• To determine if there is sciatic nerve root compression	• Forward bending in standing causes the affected knee to flex if the test is positive	• If the patient is not permitted to flex the knee, then lumbar flexion is less	• SLR is usually also positive • More sensitive if unilateral • Rule out hamstrings

SLUMP TEST

Purpose	Positive Test	Interpretation	Comments
• To reproduce the patient's low back and/or leg symptoms	• The patient flexes the spine while sitting, maintaining the neck in neutral, then flexes the head with overpressure, followed by knee extension and foot dorsiflexion, ending with head extension. The test is positive if these maneuvers reproduce the patient's symptoms	• Indicates increased tension in the neuromeningeal tract (disc lesion, dural stretching)	• If symptoms are reproduced at any stage, continuing the test is not indicated • May also extend both legs • Use only if other provocation tests are negative when neural compromise is suspected

STORK EXTENSION TEST

Purpose	Positive Test	Interpretation	Comments
• This may determine if there is spondylolisthesis	• The patient stands on one leg and extends the trunk	• If positive, there is pain in the back	• May indicate a stress fracture at the pars

PHEASANT TEST

Purpose	Positive Test	Interpretation	Comments
• To determine if there is an unstable lumbar segment	• A positive test is present when pain arises while applying pressure to the patient's lumbar spine while you flex the knees in prone	• Indicates an unstable segment	• If positive, avoid any further lumbar extension

SPRING TEST

Purpose	Positive Test	Interpretation	Comments
• To assess segmental mobility and quality of joint play; can also help determine the level of dysfunction if symptoms arise from the lumbar spine	• Apply posterior-anterior pressure to each vertebral segment at the spinous process in short quick pushes while the patient is prone and compare the segments to each other	• If there is pain or resistance to the "spring," it indicates the level of the lesion. Increased motion indicates hypermobility and decreased motion, hypomobility	• May be performed throughout the vertebral column • Avoid in cases of spondylolisthesis or instability

─── N O T E S ───

BICYCLE TEST (OF VAN GELDEREN)

Purpose	Positive Test	Interpretation	Comments
• To determine if there is neurogenic claudication (lumbar spinal stenosis)	• A positive test occurs when the patient pedals while in slight lumbar extension and leg symptoms begin, then leans forward while pedaling until symptoms decrease	• This means the radicular pain and paresthesias originate in the lumbar spine, usually from stenosis, and is not due to intermittent vascular claudication, in which case the symptoms would stay unchanged with any trunk position	• This is a very diagnostic test • Confirm also by checking pedal pulse, as both conditions may coexist

Notes

WADDELL'S TESTING

Purpose	*Positive Test*	*Interpretation*	*Comments*
• To determine if the patient is malingering • See Appendix C	• Apply 2# of head pressure • Have patient do simulated trunk rotation • Assess for tenderness to light touch in low back • Assess straight leg raising in supine, which should also be positive with knee extension in sitting • Assess for non-anatomical dermatomal or myotomal symptom distribution	• If one or more of these are present, it may indicate exaggerated pain behaviors	• Also look for subjective symptoms like whole leg pain and numbness, pain at the tip of the tail bone, ER admittance due to pain, and inability to tolerate therapy • As the number of symptoms accumulate, the more the patient may be exaggerating

─── N O T E S ───

CHAPTER EIGHT

SACROILIAC AND ILIOSACRAL DISORDERS AND SPECIAL TESTS

FORWARD SACRAL TORSION (LEFT ON LEFT [L ON L])

Characteristics	Signs and Symptoms	Special Tests	Intervention
• Most common SIJ dysfunction • Right piriformis is contracted and pulls the right sulcus forward • Sacrum is stuck, flexed anteriorly on the right • Sacral base is rotated anteriorly to the left • Sacrum is positioned in left sidebending (LSB) and left rotation (LROT) • Can be due to a short left leg, trauma, or right gluteus medius weakness	• Unilateral lumbosacral and gluteal pain • May cause sciatica • Pain with ambulation, going up stairs, and prolonged standing • Left hip usually in ER in supine • Increased lordosis • Signs are opposite for right on right (R on R)	• Posterior superior iliac spine (PSIS) is posterior on the left • Sitting forward flexion test (FFT) is positive usually on the opposite side (R) • Left sacral sulcus is shallow • Inferior lateral angle (ILA) is posterior and inferior on the left • Piriformis and tensor fascia lata (TFL) tender on opposite side	• Resist left piriformis • Direct technique for right sacral SB and right sacral rotation • Heel lift if leg length disparity • Strengthening, especially gluteus medius and maximus • Muscle energy techniques

———————— N O T E S ————————

BACKWARD SACRAL TORSION (RIGHT ON LEFT [R ON L])

Characteristics	Signs and Symptoms	Special Tests	Intervention
• Sacral base is rotated to the right • Piriformis is often the culprit • May be due to trauma	• Right PSIS is posterior • Sitting FFT is positive on right • Anterior superior iliac spine (ASIS) may be posterior and superior on the right • Right hip is in slight ER • Right sulcus is shallow • ILA is posterior and inferior on the right • Piriformis is tight and tender on the right • Decreased lordosis	• Based on signs	• Resist right hip abduction while in slight hip flexion • Direct technique • Muscle energy techniques

——————— N O T E S ———————

ANTERIOR INNOMINATE ROTATION (RIGHT)

Characteristics	Signs and Symptoms	Special Tests	Intervention
• Ilium is rotated forward • Can be due to golf, weak abdominals, gluteus medius and maximus • Pain is usually more diffuse	• Pain on lumbosacral and gluteal area, especially with gait and stairs • Tenderness to palpation on ILA and right PSIS • Left TFL may be tender	• Right ASIS is low • Right PSIS is high • Positive standing FFT • Leg appears to shorten with long sitting • Right sacral sulcus is shallow • Positive SIJ compression	• Resist hip extension • Direct technique: rotate ilium posteriorly • Isometric hip adduction after correction and strengthening exercises • "Shot-gun" technique • SI belt

POSTERIOR INNOMINATE ROTATION (LEFT)

Characteristics	Signs and Symptoms	Special Tests	Intervention
• Ilium is rotated backward • Can be due to prolonged LE weight-bearing on the left, due to fall on left ischium, left weak gluteus medius, left hamstring tightness or a short left leg, kicking, or missing a step • Pain is usually more localized	• Pain on the left lumbosacral and gluteal area with or without sciatica, especially with gait and climbing stairs • Right piriformis and/or TFL may be tender	• Left PSIS is inferior and posterior • Left ASIS is superior and anterior • Positive standing FFT • Leg appears to lengthen with long sitting • Left sulcus deep	• Resist hip flexion on the left • Direct technique: rotate left iliac bone anteriorly • Isometrics to hip adductors when corrected • "Shot-gun" technique • SI belt • Sclerosing injections if rotations do not stay corrected

INFLARE (LEFT)

Characteristics	Signs and Symptoms	Special Tests	Intervention
• Ilium is rotated inward • Usually due to muscle imbalances • Can occur with anterior ilium rotations and due to trauma or decreased hip ROM	• Diffuse pain on left lumbosacral and gluteal region, especially with unilateral stance or crossed-leg sitting • Increased piriformis tone on the left • Weakness on the left gluteus medius • Tender to palpate	• Left ilium is closer to the umbilicus • Standing FFT is positive on left • ASIS is medial on the left • PSIS is lateral • Sulcus is wider on the left	• Resist hip adduction and IR in hip flexion, abduction, and ER • Gluteus medius strengthening • Direct technique • Left piriformis stretching • Address the hip

OUTFLARE

Characteristics	Signs and Symptoms	Special Tests	Intervention
• Ilium is rotated outward • Can occur with posterior ilium rotations, hip muscle imbalances, or trauma	• Diffuse pain in lumbosacral and gluteal region • Increased piriformis tone on affected side	• Findings are opposite from inflare • Decreased hip IR on affected side	• Resist hip abduction with the hip in flexion, adduction, and IR • Piriformis stretching

UPSLIP (RIGHT)

Characteristics	Signs and Symptoms	Special Tests	Intervention
• Ilium is positioned superiorly • Usually due to a fall on the ischium or landing on one leg • Tightness on hip adductors • Not a very common finding	• Pain on the SIJ area, especially with weight-bearing • May have tenderness of right quadratus lumborum	• Standing FFT is positive on the right • ASIS and PSIS are up on the right • Right lower extremity (RLE) is short • Sulcus is shallow on right • Positive Gillet's on the right • Supine-to-sit test positive short to long	• Right long axis distraction in IR and abduction • Quadratus lumborum and hip adductor stretches • Inferior iliac glide

DOWNSLIP (LEFT)

Characteristics	Signs and Symptoms	Special Tests	Intervention
• Ilium is positioned inferiorly • Usually due to short left leg, weakness on gluteus medius, and/or tightness on left iliotibial band (ITB) • Less common than upslip	• Pain on left lumbosacral and gluteal region, especially during weight-bearing on affected side • Tender on left SIJ	• Standing FFT is positive on the left • ASIS and PSIS are down on the left • Positive Gillet's on the left • Pubic bone low on the left • Left leg may appear longer	• Quadratus lumborum and hip adductor strengthening • "Shot-gun" technique • Superior iliac glide • Left ITB stretch • Heel lift if needed

SPECIAL TESTS

STANDING FORWARD FLEXION TEST

Purpose	Positive Test	Interpretation	Comments
• To determine hypomobility of the ilia on the sacrum	• Place your thumbs on each PSIS; a positive test is shown if one PSIS moves upward with one thumb during standing trunk flexion	• Indicates that the side that moves up has restricted mobility	• Usually means that that is the side of the lesion • Also called Vorlauf phenomenon

SITTING FORWARD FLEXION TEST

Purpose	Positive Test	Interpretation	Comments
• To determine hypomobility of the sacrum on the ilia	• A positive test is shown if one PSIS moves upward with your thumb during sitting forward flexion	• Indicates that the side that moves up has restricted mobility	• Usually means that is the side of the lesion • This position eliminates hamstring involvement and stabilizes the ilia • Also called Piedallu's sign

——— N O T E S ———

SUPINE TO SIT TEST

Purpose	Positive Test	Interpretation	Comments
• To determine if there is abnormal biomechanics of the ilium resulting in an apparent leg length discrepancy	• A positive test results when one medial malleoli appears to lengthen or shorten as the patient does a long sit-up, while your thumbs are monitoring the malleoli at the foot of the plinth	• A short-to-long leg indicates there is a posterior ilium rotation • A long-to-short leg indicates an anterior ilium rotation	• The side that changes length usually correlates with the involved side of the standing forward flexion test

GILLET'S TEST

Purpose	Positive Test	Interpretation	Comments
• To determine hypomobility	• The test is positive if one PSIS does not move downward while the patient stands with one hip fully flexed and your thumbs are on both PSISs (stork position)	• Indicates restrictions on the side that does not move or moves very little • The previous four tests are more valid if at least three are positive	• This test also usually correlates with the involved side of the standing FFT • Also called stork test or sacral fixation test

SACROILIAC (SI) GAP AND COMPRESSION TESTS

Purpose	Positive Test	Interpretation	Comments
• To determine if the pain is of SI origin	• A positive test occurs when there is SIJ pain as you approximate or separate the ilia, while the patient is supine	• Indicates anterior SI ligament sprain if there is pain during separation (gapping) and posterior SI lesion if there is pain with ilia approximation (compression)	• May perform compression test one ilium at a time in sidelying • These terms refer to the pelvic motion and not the joint motion, as one test gaps one area of the joint while compressing the other

SQUISH TEST

Purpose	Positive Test	Interpretation	Comments
• To test for the integrity of the posterior SI ligaments	• Pain will arise if the test is positive while you push the anterior ilia down and in at a 45 degree angle while the patient is supine	• Indicates a sprain on the posterior SI ligaments	• This test may not be needed if the SI gapping test was positive

HIBB'S TEST

Purpose	Positive Test	Interpretation	Comments
• To test for the integrity of the posterior SI ligaments	• Internally rotate the hip while at 90 degrees of knee flexion in prone and palpate the ipsilateral SI joint	• Compare both sides to assess the degree of joint "opening"	• Pain with this may indicate the posterior SI joint is involved • Also known as prone gapping test

CHAPTER NINE

HIP AND THIGH DISORDERS AND SPECIAL TESTS

DEGENERATIVE JOINT DISEASE

Characteristics	Signs and Symptoms	Special Tests	Intervention
• Can be primary (due to aging) or secondary (due to previous problems) • Most common disease of the hip • Usually of gradual onset in adults older than 40 • More common in women than in men	• Pain is located around the groin and rarely referred below the knee • Morning stiffness <30 minutes • Aching, especially at night and with activity • Gait deviations • Capsular tightness • Limited ROM and function	• Positive scour test • Positive grind test • Positive Faber's test • Positive Thomas' test • Decreased ROM • Hypomobility • X-ray (osteophytes)	• Medication • Joint mobilization and ROM exercises • Decrease stress to hip (weight loss) • Stretching exercises • Use adaptive equipment: cane, elevated seats • Hip abductor strengthening • Surgery: total hip replacement (THR)

MUSCLE STRAINS AND TEARS

Characteristics	Signs and Symptoms	Special Tests	Intervention
• Usually due to poor stretching, muscle imbalance, and overuse • Can cause avulsion fractures • Pain is sudden or occurs right after a sporting event • Usually on hamstrings, rectus femoris, adductor longus, psoas, and sartorius muscles	• Tenderness to palpation • Swelling • Bruising • Pain with passive stretching and AROM • Tissue texture abnormalities	• Pain with resisted isolated motions • Local tenderness • History	• PRICE if acute • Decreased weight-bearing • DFM if tolerated after the acute stage • US • Progress to stretching, strengthening, and eccentric training avoiding pain, closed kinetic chain (CKC), and plyometric exercises

TROCHANTERIC BURSITIS

Characteristics	Signs and Symptoms	Special Tests	Intervention
• Inflamed bursae at the greater trochanter • Can occur from biomechanical problems (leg length discrepancy), pressure, or trauma • ITB can snap over the greater trochanter, especially in runners • Common in women • Ischial and iliopectineal bursitis are less common	• Onset of pain is insidious, located on the lateral hip, and can refer to L5 dermatome, especially going up stairs, sidelying, and getting out of a car • ROM is usually complete, but adduction can be limited	• Pain with resisted abduction and IR/ER • Positive Ober's test • Localized tenderness to palpation	• US • Abductor stretching exercises • Hip pads • Pillow between knees • Avoid aggravators • Cortisone injections

HIP POINTER

Characteristics	Signs and Symptoms	Special Tests	Intervention
• Contusion on the iliac crest, ASIS, or both • Can cause avulsion fracture (sartorius) • Common in athletes (helmet strike)	• Localized pain to iliac crest	• Tenderness • Mechanism of injury	• Iontophoresis • Ice • Hip stretching exercises • Protective gear

MERALGIA PARESTHETICA

Characteristics	Signs and Symptoms	Special Tests	Intervention
• Known as lateral femoral cutaneous nerve entrapment • Can be due to trauma, pressure (truss, tool belt), obesity, leg length discrepancy (LLD), L2 to L3 DDD or HNP, short leg on the opposite side, diabetes, and pregnancy • Nerve is entrapped at the ASIS where the nerve passes through the inguinal ligament	• Pain is of gradual or sudden onset affecting the anterior lateral thigh • Pain is burning and aggravated with hip adduction and forced flexion • Hypesthesia and occasional numbness • ROM usually full except for tightness and may be painful at end range • Tenderness to palpate	• Positive neurologic signs if nerve root is involved • Positive prone knee bend test • NCV	• Pain modalities • Patient education (weight loss, remove tool belt, etc) • Hip extension exercises • Treat lumbar spine if involved • Gentle lower limb stretching • May need a heel lift • Nerve blocks if severe

N O T E S

MYOSITIS OSSIFICANS

Characteristics	Signs and Symptoms	Special Tests	Intervention
• Calcium deposition from a contusion resulting from a direct blow to the thigh, either repeated or from a single trauma • Can also occur in the arm and elbow • Do not confuse with heterotopic ossification (osteoblastic activity) seen in traumatic brain injury, spinal cord injury, total hip replacement, and coma	• Local pain at the site of the contusion • Limited knee ROM, especially flexion • May palpate tissue texture abnormalities	• Palpation for a mass (calcification) • Imaging	• In acute phase (as calcification is forming), heat and stretching are contraindicated • Ice • Maintain comfortable knee flexion • Iontophoresis with acetic acid, magnesium, or dyphosphorate • Cortisone shots, aspiration, or surgery

——————— N O T E S ———————

LEGG-CALVÉ-PERTHES DISEASE

Characteristics	Signs and Symptoms	Special Tests	Intervention
• Decreased blood flow to the femur: osteo-necrosis • Idiopathic but may be familial, due to trauma or low birth weight • More common in white boys (4:1) between 2 and 13 years of age • Incidence is 1 in 1200 • Usually unilateral • Can cause problems later in life • Has four stages and is self-limiting	• Gradual onset of pain in the hip, groin, thigh, and knee, especially with weight-bearing • Tenderness to palpation • Decreased abduction, internal rotation, and extension • Trendelenburg gait • Muscle spasms • Decreased functional activities	• X-ray	• Bed rest • Weight-bearing in abduction splint • Abduction and IR splint • Leg traction

———— N O T E S ————

SLIPPED CAPITAL FEMORAL EPIPHYSIS

Characteristics	Signs and Symptoms	Special Tests	Intervention
• May be due to trauma, obesity, or increased growth hormone • Usually unilateral in 10- to 17-year-old boys on the left side • Can cause problems later in life	• Mild pain to palpation in the hip, pelvis, thigh, and knee in chronic cases • LLD • Quadriceps atrophy • Decreased ROM, especially IR, abduction, and flexion • Trendelenburg gait	• X-ray (displaced upper femoral epiphysis)	• Limit weight-bearing • Rest • Splinting • Usually corrected with surgery

CONGENITAL HIP DISLOCATION

Characteristics	Signs and Symptoms	Special Tests	Intervention
• Also known as developmental dysplasia of the hip • Occurs at birth with an 8:1 female to male ratio • Mostly in whites and on the left side • May come with acetabular or femoral dysplasia and anteversion • Incidence is 1 in 1000	• Decreased abduction • Leg held in flexion with abduction	• Positive Galeazzi's, telescoping, and Ortolani's signs (usually done by MD) • X-ray	• Splints to maintain reduction of the dislocation (frog position) • Surgery • The last five conditions may require gait training

TOTAL HIP ARTHROPLASTY

Characteristics	Signs and Symptoms	Special Tests	Intervention
• Most common hip procedure • More common in older women • Usually due to DJD • Indicated for severe hip pain, limited motion, and weight-bearing, resulting in limited function	• Usually very painful after surgery • Limited mobility and strength	• Surgical • May include trochanteric osteotomy, in which case gait and active exercises to involved muscles may be limited for the first 6 to 8 weeks	• Based on approach and MD • Observe hip precautions: avoid adduction and flexion past 90 degrees; for posterolateral approach, avoid also IR and ER for anterolateral approach • If cemented: gait is first partial weight-bearing (PWB) • If press fit: non-weight-bearing (NWB)

—————— N o t e s ——————

SPECIAL TESTS

SIGN OF THE BUTTOCK

Purpose	Positive Test	Interpretation	Comments
• To determine if the origin of the pain is from the buttock, lumbar spine, or the hamstrings	• While supine, do an SLR; if restricted, bend the knee	• If hip flexion does not improve, then the problem is in the buttock, indicating a positive test. If bending the knee increases hip flexion, then the problem is in the lumbar spine or hamstrings	• If positive, there is usually a non-capsular pattern of hip joint limitation and may be indicative of more serious pathology

PATRICK'S TEST

Purpose	Positive Test	Interpretation	Comments
• To identify if the symptoms come from the hip, the lumbar region, or the SIJ	• Hip pathology, usually osteoarthritis, is indicated if there is pain while placing the patient's leg in a figure 4 position while supine	• Pain in the lumbar spine indicates a lumbar lesion, and SIJ pain indicates pathology in that joint	• There may be tightness and restricted mobility, but if this is nonpainful, the test can be considered negative, unless the restriction is severe (Jansen's test) • Also known as Faber's test for the position of the hip (flexion, abduction, and external rotation)

SCOURING TEST

Purpose	Positive Test	Interpretation	Comments
• To identify if symptoms come from the hip	• The test is positive if symptoms occur while the patient's hip is flexed, adducted, and the knee flexed, while you internally rotate the hip and compress the knee into the hip, then abduct and externally rotate the joint to "scour" it	• Indicates degenerative changes in the hip joint • May also indicate acetabular labrum tear especially if there is tenderness posterior to the greater trochanter	• Must be done with care • The patient is supine • Also known as quadrant test for the hip

GRIND TEST

Purpose	Positive Test	Interpretation	Comments
• To determine if there are degenerative changes in the joint	• With the patient supine and hip flexed to 90 degrees, apply downward pressure with rotation to the knee with your sternum or hands in an attempt to grind the joint. A positive test will result in pain	• Indicates altered joint surfaces, usually due to degenerative problems	• The applied rotation is arthrokinematic • May be performed on other joints • May feel crepitus

ANVIL TEST

Purpose	Positive Test	Interpretation	Comments
• To identify if there is a lower extremity fracture or severe hip pathology	• Localized pain to a specific area will occur when you punch the patient's elevated heel while supine	• Indicates a fracture in the calcaneus if the pain is localized there, or in the tibia or femur if these sites are the painful ones	• If lower extremity elevation is not possible, it may be done in neutral hip position

—— N O T E S ——

CHAPTER TEN

KNEE DISORDERS
AND
SPECIAL TESTS

MEDIAL COLLATERAL LIGAMENT SPRAIN/TEAR

Characteristics	Signs and Symptoms	Special Tests	Intervention
• Common in skiers and football players • More common than a lateral collateral ligament (LCL) sprain • Usually due to direct blow to the lateral knee and to side cuts (valgus stress and ER of the tibia) • May be accompanied by other medial tissue tears • Grade I: tenderness, mild sprain with minimal tissue damage (0- to 5-mm opening) • Grade II: partial tear with some laxity (5- to 10-mm opening) • Grade III: complete tear with instability (empty end feel 10 or more mm opening)	• Pain • Limited knee flexion and extension • Swelling • Tenderness to palpation at the site of the sprain or tear • Altered gait pattern • May develop thigh weakness	• Positive valgus stress test • Positive Apley's distraction with rotation • If other tissues are involved, specific tests will be positive	• PRICE with ES in acute and subacute stages • Bracing • Partial weight-bearing 2 to 3 weeks • US progressed from pulsed to continuous duty cycle as healing occurs • Early knee ROM in the brace • Progress to gentle PROM, especially flexion after 3 weeks • Progress to strengthening and functional exercises, especially quadriceps (quads) • Grade III results in surgery if above conservative approach fails (NWB 3 weeks, brace at 45-degree flexion, and isometrics)

LATERAL COLLATERAL LIGAMENT SPRAIN/TEAR

Characteristics	Signs and Symptoms	Special Tests	Intervention
• See medial collateral ligament (MCL) grades • Usually entails a blow to the medial side of the knee • May involve the ITB and/or the biceps femoris loosening from their attachments • May be accompanied by anterior cruciate ligament (ACL) and/or meniscal injuries	• Swelling • Tenderness to palpation at the site of the sprain or tear • Altered gait • Pain • Limited ROM • May develop thigh weakness	• Positive varus stress test • If other tissues are involved, specific tests will be positive	• See MCL approach • Heals slower than MCL • Complete tears usually need surgery

——————— N O T E S ———————

ACL Sprain (Deficiency)

Characteristics	Signs and Symptoms	Special Tests	Intervention
• See grades for MCL sprain • Usually due to sports like soccer • Mechanisms: hyperextension injury, lower extremity IR with body in ER, deceleration injury, anterior force on the tibia with the knee at 90 degrees and/or valgus and varus forces • A loud "pop" is usually heard	• Mild pain if completely torn • Swelling • Buckling • May have limited ROM • Feeling of instability • May develop thigh weakness • Joint hypermobility	• Positive Lachman's test • Positive anterior drawer test • Positive Slocum test • Positive MacIntosh test • Positive valgus test • Mechanism of injury • KT 1000	• Bracing • If deficient, focus on hamstring strengthening • If reconstructed, based on surgical technique and MD • Treatment should include patellar mobilizations

PCL Sprain

Characteristics	Signs and Symptoms	Special Tests	Intervention
• See grades for MCL • Usually due to trauma (dashboard injury or fall on tibial tuberosity, severe hyperextension, or hyperflexion)	• Usually no "pop" • Pain, especially with flexion • Instability • May develop thigh weakness	• Positive posterior drawer sign • Positive Hughston's tests • Positive sag sign • Positive varus and valgus stress tests	• Focus on quad strengthening • Bracing • Basic knee rehabilitation • Surgery

QUAD OR PATELLAR TENDINITIS (JUMPER'S KNEE)

Characteristics	Signs and Symptoms	Special Tests	Intervention
• Inflammation usually due to occupational or sports overuse (volleyball, basketball) • Can be due to biomechanical alterations or from not warming up • Common in adolescent athletes, or in 20- to 40-year-olds, especially on the inferior pole of patella • Grade I: pain after activity • Grade II: pain during and after activity • Grade III: pain limits activity • Grade IV: rupture	• Pain with weight-bearing activities, especially running and jumping • Resisted extension reproduces symptoms • Painful palpation on tendinous insertion, above or below the patella • AROM is painful and slightly decreased • Weakness • Localized swelling • May develop atrophy and fibrosis • Tissue texture abnormalities	• Resisted extension reproduces pain • Based on signs and symptoms	• Avoid aggravators • Medication • Phonophoresis or iontophoresis • Ice • Deep friction massage or augmented soft tissue mobilization • Quad stretching • Gradual strengthening • Tendon compression/bracing/orthotics if needed • Patellar mobilizations

——————— N O T E S ———————

QUAD OR PATELLAR TENDON RUPTURE

Characteristics	Signs and Symptoms	Special Tests	Intervention
• Usually occurs at 90 degrees of flexion due to trauma or overuse, especially in weightlifters • Common in older adults with tight quads due to falls	• Quad tendon tear may show a gap above the patella in acute stages • Unable to actively extend the knee • Pain at the site of the rupture • Swelling • Decreased weight-bearing ability	• Based on history, signs, and symptoms • Imaging	• Surgery • Postsurgically: gradual ROM exercises • Gradual weight-bearing • Gradual strengthening • Soft tissue work • Patellar mobilizations

PATELLAR BURSITIS

Characteristics	Signs and Symptoms	Special Tests	Intervention
• Most common is prepatellar bursitis: "housemaid's knee" due to prolonged kneeling • May occur from trauma • Common in wrestlers and surfers	• Swelling or puffiness • May have a callus • Tenderness to palpate • May be asymptomatic • ROM usually full but tight with overpressure into flexion	• Based on signs and symptoms	• Ice if acute • Heat later stages • US • Use knee pads • Aspiration or excision if more severe

PES ANSERINE BURSITIS

Characteristics	Signs and Symptoms	Special Tests	Intervention
• Usually due to occupational or sports overuse (running) or a direct blow • May have a biomechanical component • May be accompanied by tendinitis • Onset is usually gradual	• Pain and tenderness at the site of the bursae • Can be reproduced with resisted hip flexion, external or internal rotation, abduction, and with palpation • May have slightly decreased AROM	• Based on signs and symptoms	• Phonophoresis or iontophoresis • Ice • Limitation of aggravators • Address foot and ankle if there are biomechanical deficits

PLICA SYNDROME

Characteristics	Signs and Symptoms	Special Tests	Intervention
• Plica is a normal variation of a band of tissue from synovial recess • Usually initiated by trauma • More common in joggers and swimmers	• Pain, usually along the medial patella • Swelling, especially on the superior-medial aspect of the patella • Pseudolocking and snapping	• Palpation • Imaging • Positive mediopatellar plica test	• US and ice • Mobilizations • Stretching quads and hamstrings • Strengthening same if weak • Brace/surgery

ILIOTIBIAL BAND (ITB) FRICTION SYNDROME

Characteristics	Signs and Symptoms	Special Tests	Intervention
• Irritation at the lateral femoral condyle: ITB snaps over it from extension to flexion • Usually due to sports overuse, especially running downhill and biking, change in sporting patterns (terrain, shoes) • May cause patellofemoral syndrome • May be due to biomechanical problems: anteversion, pronation, pes cavus, and knee varus • Onset is usually gradual	• Pain on lateral knee, especially during sporting activity • Pain may radiate up or down • Lateral thigh/knee tightness • Tenderness to palpation 2 cm above the joint • There may be crepitus with knee flexion and extension	• Positive Ober's test • Positive Noble's test	• US • Deep friction massage • Lateral hip and knee stretching, including lateral retinaculum • Increase quad strength, especially VMO • Modification of sports • Hydrocortisone shots • Orthotics • Avoid running/biking for 6 weeks • Surgical release

N O T E S

MENISCAL TEARS

Characteristics	Signs and Symptoms	Special Tests	Intervention
• Can occur due to twisting and rotation, especially in soccer • Two types: peripheral tears and body tears (bucket handle) • Small tears may heal • More common on medial meniscus • May cause osteoarthritis and instability	• Pain at the joint line • Locking • Buckling • Inability to fully extend or flex the knee • Swelling • Pain with weight-bearing • Quad atrophy imaging positive • Joint popping may be present	• Positive McMurray's test • Positive Apley's test • Positive Payr's test	• PRICE in acute stages • Open kinetic chain exercises progressing to closed chain exercises • Most tears require surgery

UNHAPPY TRIAD (O'DONOGHUE)

Characteristics	Signs and Symptoms	Special Tests	Intervention
• MCL, ACL, and peripheral medial meniscus tears • Usually due to forces with the knee in slight flexion, tibial ER, and valgus and anterior translation of the tibia on the femur • Often seen in football players	• Pain • Inability to bear weight • Swelling • Decreased ROM • Atrophy • Weakness • Tenderness to palpation • Instability	• Imaging • Based on mechanism of injury, signs, and symptoms	• PRICE • Bracing • Surgery, with treatment based on surgical technique and MD • Patellar mobilizations and strengthening • ES for swelling and/or re-education

OSTEOARTHRITIS

Characteristics	Signs and Symptoms	Special Tests	Intervention
• Can be primary or secondary • Common in obese women and older adults, usually due to biomechanical abnormalities (like leg length discrepancy) or from previous trauma (meniscal) • Progressive • Can encompass the entire knee or just one compartment	• Pain, especially with weight-bearing • Deformity (varus, valgus, or flexion) • Limited motion • May have swelling • Weakness • Morning stiffness • May have instability • Quad atrophy • Crepitus	• Positive valgus and/or varus tests • Tenderness to palpation along joint lines • X-ray (spurs, narrow joint space)	• Rest/bracing • Heat or ice • Weight loss • Assistive devices • Medication • ROM and strengthening • Aquatic therapy (unloading) • Mobilization if not unstable • Hamstring stretching • Surgery

———— N O T E S ————

OSTEOCHONDRITIS DISSECANS

Characteristics	Signs and Symptoms	Special Tests	Intervention
• Bone changes resulting in loose bodies in joint • More common on the postero-lateral aspect of the medial femoral condyle • Due to trauma, poor blood supply, or hereditary factors • Usually occurs in adolescent boys • In older patients it can lead to osteonecrosis	• Diffuse knee pain • Slight effusion • Tenderness to palpation • Quad atrophy	• Positive Wilson test • X-ray	• Rest • Surgery if there is a loose body • Basic knee rehabilitation

—————— N O T E S ——————

PATELLOFEMORAL PAIN SYNDROME

Characteristics	Signs and Symptoms	Special Tests	Intervention
• Extensor mechanism dysfunction • Classified clinically as being due to instability, malalignment, or dysfunction without malalignment • Usually due to biomechanical deficits (anteversion, femoral or tibial torsion, pronation, increased quadricep angle, joint incongruencies) • May be due to trauma, recurrent subluxations, tibiofemoral disorders, surgery, muscle imbalances, or combination • More common in young women • Usually gradual onset and may be bilateral	• Pain with prolonged sitting and when descending stairs • Minimal swelling, if at all • Altered tracking mechanism • Crepitus • Patella malaligned, usually laterally displaced or "squinting" • Pain around and under the patella, especially with flexion • There may be some buckling	• Based on signs and symptoms • Positive Clarke's test • Positive "J" sign during tracking • Positive grind test	• Stretch lateral knee structures (vastus lateralus [VL], lateral retinaculum, ITB) • Strengthen medial knee structures (vastus medialis obliquous [VMO], hip adductors) • No full arc quads • Biofeedback • Patellar taping • Address other biomechanical factors • May need orthotics

PATELLAR DISLOCATION/SUBLUXATION

Characteristics	Signs and Symptoms	Special Tests	Intervention
• More common laterally and in adolescent girls • Mechanism of injury can be due to foot planted in ER with knee flexed and in valgus with a strong quad contraction due to anatomical variations, increased Q angle, external tibial torsion, muscle imbalances, valgus knee • Can reduce spontaneously • Can be intra- or extra-articular, vertical, or horizontal • 30% of patients with acute dislocations can redislocate, especially if younger than 20 years of age	• If acute dislocation, there is intense pain and inability to move the knee • The dislocation is visible • There may be avulsion fractures on medial aspect of the patella, cartilage damage, and medial soft tissue tears • Subluxations result in tenderness, especially on medial facet and medial retinaculum • Usually hypermobile	• Positive apprehension test • X-ray (especially tangential view)	• Usually closed reduction and immobilization for 2 to 6 weeks • Weight-bearing as tolerated (WBAT) • After reduction, treatment focus is on quad strengthening • Similar treatment to patellofemoral pain syndrome

MENISCECTOMY

Characteristics	Signs and Symptoms	Special Tests	Intervention
• Surgical removal or repair of one or both menisci • More common on medial side • Usually done arthroscopically • Can be performed in combination with other repairs (ACL)	• Swelling • Pain • Limited ROM • Weakness • Atrophy • Difficulty with weight-bearing	• Surgical	• PRICE • ES for swelling and/or muscle re-education • PROM progressing to strengthening • Opened and closed kinetic chain exercises • If the meniscus was repaired (versus removed), weight-bearing is usually delayed

ACL RECONSTRUCTION

Characteristics	Signs and Symptoms	Special Tests	Intervention
• May use allograft or autograft form TFL, hamstrings, patellar tendon • Most common is bone-patellar tendon-bone graft from the central third of the tendon • Can be arthroscopically assisted or miniarthrotomy	• Swelling • Mild pain • Limited ROM • Weakness • Atrophy • Difficulty with weight-bearing • If patellar tendon was used, patellar mobility will be diminished	• Surgical	• Per physician protocol and surgical technique • Most common approach is the accelerated protocol and should include patellar mobilizations

OTHER SURGICAL PROCEDURES

Characteristics	Signs and Symptoms	Special Tests	Intervention
• May be arthroscopic, open, or combined procedures • Examples: lateral release, debridement, resurfacing, excisions, resections, open reductions with internal fixation, total knee arthroplasty, high tibial osteotomy (HTO), Maquet procedure, etc	• Similar to previous tables in differing degrees	• Surgical	• Same as previous table (focus is on decreasing swelling, increasing motion, strength, and function) based on the patient's signs and symptoms and on physician protocol • WB restrictions vary according to procedure, age, diagnosis, etc

———— N o t e s ————

SPECIAL TESTS

VALGUS TEST

Purpose	Positive Test	Interpretation	Comments
• To identify medial knee instability	• If positive, there will be pain and/or excessive movement of the tibia away from the femur while you apply an abduction force to the lower leg and stabilize the knee	• Indicates disruption of the MCL, PCL, ACL, semimembranosus, posterior oblique ligament, posterior medial capsule, and/or medial quadriceps expansion	• Does not identify the exact structure that is damaged • May also be done in 30 degrees of flexion

VARUS TEST

Purpose	Positive Test	Interpretation	Comments
• To identify lateral knee instability	• If positive, there will be pain and/or excessive motion away from the femur while applying an adduction force to the lower leg as the knee is stabilized	• Indicates disruption of the LCL, PCL, ACL, ITB, posterolateral capsule, arcuate-popliteus complex, biceps femoris tendon, and/or lateral gastrocnemius	• Does not identify the exact structure that is damaged • May also be done in 30 degrees of flexion

LACHMAN TEST

Purpose	Positive Test	Interpretation	Comments
• To identify an ACL lesion • This tests one-plane anterior instability	• If the test is positive, there will be excessive motion (>3 mm) and a soft end feel while you glide the tibia forward, stabilizing the thigh with the knee at 30 degrees of flexion and the patient supine or sitting	• Indicates ACL disruption and anterior instability • The PCL and arcuate-popliteus complex may also be injured	• This is a very sensitive test for the ACL (PL band) • Excessive motion is identified by the disappearance of infrapatellar tendon slope

POSTERIOR SAG SIGN

Purpose	Positive Test	Interpretation	Comments
• To identify a PCL lesion	• If the test is positive, the tibia will appear more posterior when the patient's legs are observed at 90 degrees of knee flexion with the feet supported in the supine position	• Indicates a disruption of the PCL	• There is posterior joint instability

SLOCUM TEST

Purpose	Positive Test	Interpretation	Comments
• To determine if there is anterio-lateral rotatory instability (ALRI)	• If the test is positive for ALRI, the tibia will move more on the lateral side as an anterior force is applied to the flexed knee (90 degrees), with flexed hip (45 degrees) and the tibia internally rotated. Stabilize the foot by sitting on it	• Indicates ALRI • If the test is done with the tibia in external rotation, a positive test would indicate anterior medial instability	• The ACL is usually affected if these are positive • The patient should be supine

MACINTOSH TEST

Purpose	Positive Test	Interpretation	Comments
• To determine if there is anterior rotatory instability	• Apply a valgus stress with the knee extended and internally rotated as you flex the knee. The test is positive if at 30 to 40 degrees of flexion there is a sudden jump on the lateral tibial plateau	• Denotes ALRI • The jump is due to the tibia subluxing on the femur, then reducing	• The ACL is usually affected if the test is positive • Also called lateral pivot shift test

HUGHSTON'S POSTEROMEDIAL DRAWER TEST

Purpose	Positive Test	Interpretation	Comments
• To determine if there is posterior medial rotatory instability	• A positive test results when the tibia moves excessively or rotates posteriorly when a posterior force is applied as the lower leg is internally rotated while flexed to 45 degrees and stabilized in supine by sitting on the patient's foot	• Indicates that the PCL, MCL, posterior medial capsule, posterior oblique ligament, semimembranosus muscle, and ACL may be disrupted	• The test may also be performed with the patient sitting, while the therapist stabilizes the lower extremity with his or her legs

HUGHSTON'S POSTEROLATERAL DRAWER TEST

Purpose	Positive Test	Interpretation	Comments
• To determine if there is posterior lateral rotatory instability	• A positive test results when the tibia moves excessively or rotates posteriorly when a posterior force is applied as the lower leg is externally rotated (stabilizing as noted in previous table)	• Indicates a PCL tear, but there may also be tears of LCL, biceps tendon, arcuate-popliteus complex, ACL, and posterolateral capsule	• The test may also be performed with the patient sitting as previously mentioned

McMurray's Test

Purpose	Positive Test	Interpretation	Comments
• To determine if there is a meniscal lesion, usually on the posterior horn	• A positive test is noted if there is crepitus or clicking over the joint line as the flexed knee is extended, while external and internal rotational forces are applied to the tibia and the joint line is palpated in supine. A valgus force may also be applied during the maneuver	• If there is clicking in external rotation, the medial meniscus is affected, and if in internal rotation, the lateral meniscus is injured	• The test is usually painful, and the more extended the leg is while the click is felt, the more posterior the lesion

Payr's Test

Purpose	Positive Test	Interpretation	Comments
• To identify a meniscal injury	• A positive sign is present when there is pain on the medial side of the joint line as the patient's leg is placed in a figure 4 position while supine	• Usually the posterior horn of the medial meniscus is affected	• May also be tested while sitting "indian style" and applying downward pressure on the involved knee

APLEY'S TEST

Purpose	Positive Test	Interpretation	Comments
• To see if there is a meniscal injury with compression or a ligamentous injury with distraction	• While prone at 90 degrees of knee flexion, rotate the tibia in both directions with distraction then compression	• The test is positive for meniscal injury if rotation and compression cause pain	• Look for hypo-, hypermobility, and/or pain

MEDIOPATELLAR PLICA TEST

Purpose	Positive Test	Interpretation	Comments
• To determine if the plica is being impinged between the medial femoral condyle and the patella	• A positive test results in pain as the patella is moved medially with the knee flexed up to 30 degrees	• Indicates an irritable plica	• May be done in supine or sitting

BALLOTABLE TEST

Purpose	Positive Test	Interpretation	Comments
• To determine if there is swelling in the knee joint	• A positive sign is felt when the knee cap "floats" as slight pressure or tapping is done on its surface	• Indicates joint effusion	• May be done with the knee extended or slightly bent • Also known as patellar tap test

CLARKE'S TEST

Purpose	Positive Test	Interpretation	Comments
• To determine if there is patellofemoral pain syndrome	• Exists when there is pain and inability to maintain a contraction as a downward and inferior pressure is applied with the web of the therapist's hand to the suprapatellar area while the patient attempts to contract the quadriceps	• Indicates retropatellar pain	• This is performed while the knee is in extension, but different degrees of flexion may be needed to test other retropatellar areas • Also called patellofemoral grind test

APPREHENSION TEST

Purpose	Positive Test	Interpretation	Comments
• To determine if the patella is prone to dislocate	• The patient will show signs of apprehension and contract the quadriceps in response to a careful lateral glide of the patella while the knee is placed in 30 degrees of flexion	• The test is usually performed in cases of recurrent dislocation	• The patient feels the knee cap will dislocate • Must be done with caution

NOBEL'S COMPRESSION TEST

Purpose	Positive Test	Interpretation	Comments
• To ascertain whether there is an ITB syndrome	• A positive test results in pain at 30 degrees when the patient's knee is passively extended from 90 degrees, while pressure is applied just proximally to the lateral femoral epicondyle	• Indicates ITB irritation	• This is considered a good diagnostic test

WILSON TEST

Purpose	Positive Test	Interpretation	Comments
• To determine if there is osteochondritis dissecans	• Extend the flexed knee while internally rotating the tibia. Pain increases at 30 degrees of flexion, at which point externally rotate the tibia. If the pain disappears, this indicates a positive sign.	• This is only true if the defect is located on the medial femoral condyle	• Must differentiate with rotatory and meniscal lesions

CHAPTER ELEVEN

ANKLE DISORDERS
AND
SPECIAL TESTS

ACUTE LATERAL ANKLE SPRAINS/TEARS

Characteristics	Signs and Symptoms	Special Tests	Intervention
• Complete or partial rupture of anterior talofibular (ATF), calcaneofibular (CF), and/or posterior talofibular (PTF) ligaments, and/or the deltoid ligament if there is a medial sprain • 80% are inversion sprains • Three grades or stages according to mechanism of injury, position of the foot, or number of ligaments involved • Can also result in avulsion fractures	• Grade I: pain and swelling on anterolateral aspect of lateral malleolus, point tenderness, and no laxity • Grade II: tearing, popping on lateral aspect, pain and swelling, tenderness, positive anterior drawer test, and may involve more ligaments • Grade III: grade II plus complete tear of the ligament(s), diffuse swelling, ecchymosis, and increased pain with difficulty weight-bearing; may be accompanied by fractures	• Based on signs, symptoms, and mechanism of injury • Positive anterior and posterior drawer tests • Positive talar tilt test • X-ray	• Medication • Grades 1 and 2: PRICE, pulsed US, crutches, painfree ROM and biomechanical ankle platform system (BAPS [Spectrum Therapy Products, Jasper, MI]), brace or taping, progressing to strengthening, especially peroneals and agility drills for athletes • Grade 3: rigid protection 1 to 3 weeks • Limit weight-bearing • Surgery for severe or recurrent cases

——————— N O T E S ———————

CHRONIC LATERAL ANKLE INSTABILITY

Characteristics	Signs and Symptoms	Special Tests	Intervention
• Recurrent ankle sprains • May include subluxation of the peroneal tendons • Can be due to decreased proprioception	• Instability on hills or uneven terrain • Hypermobility • Pain and swelling with activity • Weakness, especially peroneals	• Positive anterior drawer test • Positive talar tilt test • X-ray (stress films)	• Strengthening • Proprioception • Support • Reconstructive surgery in about 20% of patients

SEVER'S DISEASE

Characteristics	Signs and Symptoms	Special Tests	Intervention
• Calcaneal epiphysitis • More common in 10- to 15-year-olds • Occurs at the Achilles' insertion • Can occur due to trauma, but mostly from sports like running • Usually self-limiting	• Pain on the heel during activity • Tender to palpate • Tight heel cord	• X-ray	• Anti-inflammatories • Heel lift • Taping • Rest • Ice • Gradual stretching

SYNDESMOTIC SPRAINS (ANKLE DIASTASIS)

Characteristics	Signs and Symptoms	Special Tests	Intervention
• Anterior tibiofibular ligament sprain but is rare in isolation • More common with talocrural joint sprains • Usually caused by injury in dorsiflexion (DF) or plantarflexion (PF) with ER of the foot and IR of the leg, due to direct blow or uneven terrain	• Decreased ROM • Tenderness to palpation • Minimal local swelling and ecchymosis • Difficulty with weight-bearing • Palpation over distal anterior tibiofibular joint is painful	• Positive side-to-side test • Squeezing above the ankle or ER passive stress test with ankle neutral may cause pain • Stress films	• Control pain and swelling and increased painfree AROM • Protective gait • PRICE • Taping or brace • Iontophoresis or phonophoresis • BAPS • Strengthening

POSTERIOR TIBIALIS TENDINITIS

Characteristics	Signs and Symptoms	Special Tests	Intervention
• Usually a chronic degenerative inflammatory process resulting in posteromedial ankle pain • Common in women older than 40 • May be due to poor biomechanical alignment and/or excessive running • Associated with foot pronation • May progress to a rupture	• Tenderness to palpation on medial aspect of ankle • Pain with passive pronation and active supination • Pain with resisted inversion with plantarflexion that may radiate proximally • Pain is worse with walking and standing	• Based on signs and symptoms	• PRICE • Support (taping, brace, orthotics) • Phonophoresis • DFM if tolerated • Calf, posterior tibialis, and hamstring stretching • Strengthening progressing to eccentrics • If persistent, surgery for debridement and decompression

ACHILLES' TENDINITIS

Characteristics	Signs and Symptoms	Special Tests	Intervention
• Inflammation of the Achilles' tendon • Usually due to high-impact sports (running) • May be due to excessive pronation, pes cavus, tight heel cord, no warm-up, overtraining • 80% of patients are men between 30 and 50 years of age	• Pain, especially with weight-bearing activities • Swelling • Tenderness to palpation • Tendon thickening and crepitus • Pain with passive DF and resisted PF	• Based on signs and symptoms • Imaging	• PRICE • Skin roll • Heel lift, tape, or orthotics • Avoid aggravators • Gentle calf and hamstring stretching • Gradual strengthening

———— N O T E S ————

ACHILLES' TENDON RUPTURE

Characteristics	Signs and Symptoms	Special Tests	Intervention
• Sudden onset, usually due to forefoot push-off with knee extension • Common in men between 30 and 40 years of age • Usually occurs 1 to 2 inches from the heel • Can occur due to degenerative changes associated with hypovascularity and microtrauma • Misdiagnosed 25% of the time • Can rerupture in 30% of patients	• Painful "pop" • Visible defect (gap) in the tendon if seen immediately after onset and if completely torn • Decreased ROM • Inability to stand on the toes • Difficulty plantarflexing • Swelling in 1 to 2 hours • Ecchymosis	• Based on signs, symptoms, and mechanism of injury • Positive Thompson's test, especially with a complete tear	• PRICE • Surgery if complete rupture • Prolonged immobilization with or without removable cast • Post-immobilization: heel lift, gradual stretching, skin roll, DFM, heat or ice, progressing to strengthening, proprioceptive, and functional exercises

—————— N O T E S ——————

GASTROCNEMIUS TEAR

Characteristics	Signs and Symptoms	Special Tests	Intervention
• Usually partial disruption of the medial head of the gastrocnemius • Usually sudden onset while hill running, jumping, or experiencing a forceful contraction • Common during tennis, especially with DF and knee extension ("tennis leg")	• Burning pain • Hematoma • Tenderness to palpation • Tissue texture abnormalities • Tightness • Decreased weight-bearing ability • Patients feel they were shot in the leg	• Thompson's test may or may not be positive • Based on signs and symptoms	• PRICE • Heel lift • Avoid aggravators • Taping • Gentle stretching • DFM • US • Gradual strengthening after 4 weeks • Functional exercises

———— N O T E S ————

CHRONIC EXERTIONAL COMPARTMENT SYNDROME

Characteristics	Signs and Symptoms	Special Tests	Intervention
• Exercise-induced pain on the anterolateral, posteromedial, or medial aspects of the lower leg • More common on the anterolateral side • Described as overuse myositis due to exertion • Gradual onset, especially during running, and can progress to acute compartment syndrome • May be due to muscle imbalances and abnormal biomechanics (rearfoot pronation) • Usually bilateral • May occur in the foot, thigh, hand, or arm	• Pain on lower leg • Tenderness • May have some swelling/engorgement • Pain relieved with rest • If more severe, may cause numbness and tingling	• Based on signs and symptoms • Need to rule out stress fracture and acute compartment syndrome • May have increased calf circumference • Doppler • Pressure is measured with catheters or intravenous alarm control (IVAC) pump	• Rest • Ice • Stretching before and after activities • Taping in some cases • Modify sports • Good running shoes with heel counter and/or orthotics • Strengthening • Fasciotomy in severe cases

Note: Also known as shin splints.

ACUTE COMPARTMENT SYNDROME

Characteristics	Signs and Symptoms	Special Tests	Intervention
• Increased inter-compartmental pressure during exercise or due to trauma impeding blood flow (within 30 minutes) • Medical emergency	• Increasing pain • Increasing swelling that does not ease with rest • Fullness/tight skin • Numbness and tingling • Sensation loss between second and third toes • Decreased dorsalis pedis pulse	• Based on signs and symptoms	• Refer immediately to MD • Immediate ice and rest • No compression or elevation (due to increased arterial pressure) • Fasciotomy

STRESS FRACTURES

Characteristics	Signs and Symptoms	Special Tests	Intervention
• Caused by repetitive forces to the lower leg and foot (running), especially the tibia and second metatarsal bone • Pronation and a hypermobile first ray may predispose to this • Usually gradual onset over 2 to 3 weeks	• Pain • Tenderness to palpation with or without swelling • Pain with weight-bearing activities and certain movements	• Bone scan • X-ray • Pain with percussion and/or vibration • There may be pain with application of ultrasound	• Decrease activity for 1 to 3 months • Modify shoes • Surgery • Postsurgical approach focuses on decreasing swelling, increasing motion, strength, flexibility, and function

ANKLE FRACTURES

Characteristics	Signs and Symptoms	Special Tests	Intervention
• Classified based on location of fracture, position of the foot, forces applied to it, and by epiphyseal damage (Salter-Harris) • Can be uni-, bi-, or trimalleolar (both malleoli and posterior tubercle of the distal tibia) or comminuted • Some cases can result in RSD	• Pain • Swelling • Increased local temperature • Deformity • Loss of function • Inability to bear weight • Must assess proximal fibula to rule out fracture there (Maisonneuve fracture)	• X-ray • Anvil test	• Immobilization, ORIF, or external fixation • Implantable or noninvasive ES for nonunions • Treatment after healing consists of heat, ROM, mobilization, strengthening, BAPS, and open and closed kinetic chain/functional exercises • Observe for signs of RSD and treat accordingly

———— N O T E S ————

ACHILLES' TENDON REPAIR

Characteristics	Signs and Symptoms	Special Tests	Intervention
• End-to-end anastomosis • Percutaneous and subcutaneous repair • VY plasty • Tendon transfers • Some approaches entail early mobilization and others prolonged immobilization	• Swelling • Pain • Limited motion • Hypomobility • Weakness • Atrophy • Decreased proprioception • Decreased function • Decreased ambulation abilities • Full DF may be limited	• Surgical	• Postsurgical management: 6 week immobilization or early limited mobility (no DF for 6 weeks) • Heel lift • Soft tissue work • US • ES for re-education • Very gradual stretching • Gradual strengthening, especially eccentrically • Functional and proprioceptive exercises

—— N O T E S ——

ANKLE LIGAMENT RECONSTRUCTION

Characteristics	Signs and Symptoms	Special Tests	Intervention
• Various techniques: direct repair or tenodesis like the Watson-Jones, Evans, Chrisman-Snook, Broström, and anatomical, which seems to be the most successful • The peroneous brevis tendon is usually attached to the calcaneus and talus via holes through the fibula • Purpose is to provide stability and prevent inversion of the foot	• Swelling • Pain • Limited motion • Hypomobility • Weakness • Atrophy • Decreased proprioception • Decreased function • Decreased ambulation abilities	• Surgical	• Postsurgical management focuses on re-educating eversion and enhancing proprioception • Need to address swelling, decreased motion (except for inversion), and strength, as well as function

—————— NOTES ——————

SPECIAL TESTS

ANTERIOR DRAWER TEST

Purpose	Positive Test	Interpretation	Comments
• To identify injury to the anterior talofibular ligament	• With the patient prone, the distal leg is stabilized while the ankle is kept at 20 degrees of plantarflexion and the talus is pushed forward • A positive test results in increased anterior motion of the talus (with slight talar rotation)	• Indicates that the anterior talofibular ligament is disrupted • Compare with other side	• If both collateral ligaments are disrupted, the anterior translation is even (without rotation) and is better seen with the test done in dorsiflexion

POSTERIOR DRAWER TEST

Purpose	Positive Test	Interpretation	Comments
• To identify if there is an injury to the posterior talofibular ligament	• With the patient supine and the distal leg stabilized with the ankle in slight plantarflexion, mobilize the talus posteriorly and observe for excessive motion	• Indicates that the posterior talofibular ligament is sprained or torn	• If both collateral ligaments are disrupted, the posterior translation increases

TALAR TILT TEST

Purpose	Positive Test	Interpretation	Comments
• To identify if the calcaneofibular ligament is disrupted	• With the patient in sidelying, the involved side up, the ankle in neutral, and the leg stabilized, the talus is tilted side to side from abduction to adduction. Pain and/or hypermobility indicate a positive test	• An adduction force stresses the calcaneofibular ligament, and an abduction force stresses the deltoid ligament	• If possible, test the uninvolved side first for appropriate comparison of motion

SIDE-TO-SIDE TEST

Purpose	Positive Test	Interpretation	Comments
• To determine the integrity of the anterior tibiofibular ligament	• Cup the patient's heel and move the talus and calcaneus (as a unit) side to side. Increased motion compared with the uninvolved side indicates a diastasis	• Avoid tilting the talus	• The resulting motion of the maneuver is the talus hitting both malleoli from the inside of the mortise

CHAPTER TWELVE

FOOT DISORDERS
AND
SPECIAL TESTS

PLANTAR FASCIITIS

Characteristics	Signs and Symptoms	Special Tests	Intervention
• Microtears and inflammation of the plantar fascia • May be due to tight heel cord, overpronation, obesity, limited ROM of first metatarsophalangeal (MTP), high arch, and muscle imbalances • Gradual onset	• Pain, especially in the mornings, relieved in 5 to 10 minutes but worsens as day goes on • Tenderness to palpation on medial aspect of calcaneus • Pain with DF and toe extension	• Based on signs and symptoms • X-ray (may show spurs in 45% of the cases)	• PRICE • Orthotics • Taping • US • Stretching the calf and the fascia • Address first MTP joint • Dorsiflexion splint at night

TARSAL TUNNEL SYNDROME

Characteristics	Signs and Symptoms	Special Tests	Intervention
• Most common nerve entrapment of the ankle (posterior tibial nerve) • Compression is usually behind medial malleolus • May be due to chronic tendinitis, increased rearfoot pronation, or fractures	• Burning sensations and pain on the sole of the foot, especially at night and with weight-bearing • Numbness/tingling • Usually not tender on the sole of the foot	• Positive Tinel's sign • EMG/NCV • Deep tendon reflexes (DTRs) and ROM may be normal	• Rest • Orthotics • US • Heat or ice • Gentle stretching • Surgical decompression

MORTON'S NEUROMA

Characteristics	Signs and Symptoms	Special Tests	Intervention
• Metatarsalgia • More common in women between the ages of 25 and 50 • May be neurogenic, due to inappropriate shoes, tight heel cord, or poor blood supply • Usually between third and fourth metatarsals	• Burning sensation or feeling of electrical shock • Intermittent pain, especially with weightbearing • Tenderness to palpation on the site of the neuroma • Callus	• Positive compression test at MTT heads (Morton's test)	• Medication • Injections • US or phonophoresis • Iontophoresis • Shoe modification • Surgery

TURF TOE

Characteristics	Signs and Symptoms	Special Tests	Intervention
• Caused by jamming the greater toe into the end of the shoe or by hyperextending its MTP joint • Occurs frequently from running on artificial turf and by using very flexible shoes	• Pain • Tender to palpate • Swelling at the MTP joint • Ecchymosis • Difficulty and pain with push-off and passive toe extension	• Based on signs, symptoms, and mechanism of injury	• PRICE • Medication • Taping • Use of stiff-soled shoes • Sports restrictions • ROM exercises

ABNORMAL PRONATION

Characteristics	Signs and Symptoms	Special Tests	Intervention
• May be at the rearfoot, forefoot, or combined with varus in a NWB position with compensation into calcaneal valgus with weight-bearing • May be compensated or uncompensated • Associated with flattening of the medial arch • May cause or be caused by proximal and/or distal problems (tight heel cord, femoral anteversion, internal tibial torsion, knee valgus)	• May or may not be painful on the plantar aspect • Other biomechanical faults may be noted: forefoot varus, hypermobile first ray • Callus formations, especially under second metatarsal head • Can result in back pain, Achilles' tendinitis, heel spurs, plantar fasciitis, shin splints, posterior tibialis tendinitis, and patellofemoral syndrome	• Based on biomechanical alignment • Abnormal Feiss' line (navicular drop) • Foot print observation	• Gastrocnemius stretches • Better shoes • Anterior and posterior tibialis strengthening • Dynamic orthotics • Patient education • Address other components if possible

———— N O T E S ————

ABNORMAL SUPINATION

Characteristics	Signs and Symptoms	Special Tests	Intervention
• Calcaneus and/or forefoot is in varus or inversion • Classified as pes equinovarus, cavus, and cavovarus • Can lead to metatarsalgia, plantar fasciitis, stress fractures, lateral ankle sprains, and Achilles' tendinitis	• May or may not be painful on the plantar aspect • Other biomechanical faults may be noted: hypomobility of the plantar-flexed first ray • Callus formations, especially under fourth and fifth metatarsal heads	• Based on biomechanical alignment • Foot print observation	• Stretching tight muscle groups • Joint mobilization • Accommodative orthotics

——————— N o t e s ———————

SPECIAL TESTS

THOMPSON'S TEST

Purpose	Positive Test	Interpretation	Comments
• To determine if there is a rupture of the Achilles' tendon	• A positive test occurs when the patient's ankle does not plantarflex when pressure is applied to the calf muscles in prone	• Indicates a torn tendon or muscle	• The test may be negative if the strain is a grade 1 or 2 or is no longer acute

MORTON'S TEST

Purpose	Positive Test	Interpretation	Comments
• To determine if there is metatarsalgia	• A positive test results when the metatarsal heads are squeezed and the patient complains of pain or paresthesias	• Indicates a neuroma	• Some authors state that this test may also point to a stress fracture

TINEL'S SIGN

Purpose	Positive Test	Interpretation	Comments
• To determine if there is neuritis	• A positive test includes tingling and/or pain with percussion at the top of the ankle or behind the medial malleolus	• Tingling means there is regeneration • Pain and tingling means injury and degeneration	• May be positive on the anterior tibial branch of the deep peroneal nerve or posterior tibial nerve

BUERGER'S TEST

Purpose	Positive Test	Interpretation	Comments
• To determine arterial blood supply to the lower extremity	• The therapist elevates the leg to 45 degrees for 3 minutes while the patient is supine, and if the foot blanches, the test is positive, and it is confirmed when coloration returns after 1 or 2 minutes as the patient sits and dangles the legs	• Indicates decreased arterial circulation	• May correlate with intermittent vascular claudication

HOMANS' SIGN

Purpose	Positive Test	Interpretation	Comments
• To test for deep vein thrombosis	• Deep pain in the calf occurs if the test is positive and consists of dorsiflexing the ankle while squeezing the calf with the knee in extension	• Indicates poor circulation • Pain must decrease rapidly after the pressure is released for this to be indicative of thrombophlebitis	• This test may correlate with decreased pedal pulse • Swelling and pallor may also be present • Also known as Simmonds' test

CHAPTER THIRTEEN

ORTHOPAEDIC RADIOGRAPHIC EXAMINATION FOR NONPHYSICIANS

What follows is a basic description of important findings observed in orthopaedic practice. It is not intended to be an exhaustive chapter on radiology, nor is it intended to turn the physical therapist into a radiologist. Instead, it will focus on a few common structural problems and ways to examine these problems. The main objective is familiarizing the clinician with frequently used tools in the interpretation of plain films in order to enhance the patients' evaluation and management. By knowing the alignment of certain anatomical structures, we may help improve the patients' biomechanical problems (only a brief description is included on other imaging techniques).

First, when attempting to interpret a film, the clinician must make sure the image belongs to the patient in question. Therefore, it is necessary to look at the name, date, side of the film, and any other markings pertinent to the radiographic technique (ie, whether the film was taken in a weight-bearing position, at 45 degrees of flexion, etc).

Clinically, plain radiographs are usually the first study used in diagnosis, as they are less invasive and less costly than other procedures, like magnetic resonance imaging (MRI). Their importance in physical therapy is evident when, for example, after a fracture of the greater tuberosity of the humerus, a calcification that could limit abduction develops after healing. Goals for rehabilitation would thus be different from a patient who healed without a calcification, as attaining full abduction may now be unrealistic until the calcification is eliminated.

X-rays are also important because by showing joint spaces, we assess arthrokinematics to see if a decrease in the space is due to soft tissue or osseous changes (ie, the difference between therapy benefiting a patient or not).

A radiologist's findings may be negative for the condition he or she is to evaluate, and a radiologist may regard as incidental findings what physical therapists would regard as significant, such as not commenting on an impingement when assessing for humeral fractures or dislocations. This is why, in my opinion, it is valuable for us to look at the films from our perspective.

When there is little or no improvement in physical therapy and plain films have been obtained, physicians then use other procedures, such as a computerized tomography scan (CTS or CAT scan) or MRI: computer-generated slices or sections obtained through the patient. The thickness varies from 2 to 10 mm. A CAT scan shows bone better than an MRI, but it does not show soft tissue as well, and the MRI, while noninvasive, encloses the patient.

An MRI involves the response of molecules to radiation frequencies in a magnetic field. It is based on the asymmetrical distribution of charge in the nucleus of any atom. These nuclei resonate when in the field, and they absorb and emit radiofrequency energy. A computer then detects the images. Strong nuclei like hydrogen emit a strong signal. That is why, for example, normal discs appear white (on T2). Relaxation times determine the resolution of the image and are either T1 or T2. On a T1 image, fat and fluid appear black, whereas on a T2 image, they may appear white.

A bone scan or scintigraphy is used to detect changes in bone metabolism and involves the injection of a radionuclide with an affinity for bone.

Radioactive rays pass through the patient and are detected by a camera that stores data in a computer. It is an excellent detector of stress fractures but does not show pathology until 24 to 72 hours after an injury. It is also good for occult fractures, avascular necrosis, infections, and tumors.

Arthrograms, either single or double contrast, have been mostly replaced by MRIs, but they are very good at detecting soft tissue derangements like rotator cuff problems or meniscal tears.

Ultrasound is good for imaging soft tissue three-dimensionally and dynamically, and is more economical and less invasive. It is used if MRI is not more beneficial. Its sensitivity and specificity are very high. The basic principle of ultrasound is that tissues of different structures have different reflective properties. The images are obtained by electronically converting the reflective echoes and reconstructing images of the tissues through which the sound has passed.

In radiology, there are several aspects that must be observed. For example, fat lines, such as the supinator line, is seen on the lateral view of the elbow and is a thin radiolucent line parallel to the anterior aspect of the proximal one-third of the radius. It overlies the supinator muscle, separated 1 cm from the anterior margin of the radius. If elevated or widened, it may indicate joint effusion or a radial head fracture, which may not be clear on the film. Soft tissue swelling cannot be distinguished from surrounding normal tissue unless the inflammation indents, encroaches on, or obliterates fat planes.

Other x-ray characteristics include the assessment of trabecular formation. In the hip, this is measured by the Singh index for osteoporosis, which has seven grades: 7 is normal and 0 is severe osteoporosis. Another good example of cortical bone loss is the disappearance of a pedicle in the spine, but it must be differentiated from a neoplastic lesion.

Of critical importance regarding the interpretation of films is that some patients may have negative findings, yet functionally, they are wheelchair-bound. Conversely, some patients may have multiple positive findings and be perfectly functional. Therefore, the need to correlate findings on film with physical findings is of paramount importance. Recent studies, for example, have discovered that there are many asymptomatic individuals who have herniated discs or spondylolysis show up on MRI. In other words, to be valid, the findings have to match the person and be correlated with lab findings, as radiological findings are not diagnostic within themselves.

RADIOGRAPHIC EVALUATION OF COMMON SKELETAL PATHOLOGY

It is important to assess the distribution and behavior of the lesion, what bone or joint is involved, if the joint space is crossed by a lesion, if there are bony reactions, fractures, etc.

In addition, each joint has its characteristic features and measurements for assessment. To begin the examination, one assesses the ABCs of each area:

- *Alignment.* This analysis consists of assessing general skeletal structures: size, appearance, shape, deformities, cortical outline, spurs, fractures, etc.
- *Bone density.* This analysis assesses bone mineral content. One looks for thin trabeculae and local bone density changes like sclerosis, which is a sign of repair (extra bone is deposited to strengthen weight-bearing bone).
- *Cartilage space.* This analysis includes the evaluation of the width of the joint space, as cartilage is not easily visualized (due to its water content). A decreased joint space can imply degenerative cartilage or disc pathology. One also looks for erosions in subchondral bone and epiphyseal problems.
- *Soft tissues.* This analysis examines tissues by determining if there is gross swelling or atrophy, joint capsule distention by effusion, presence of gas in the tissue, calcifications, as well as fat lines.

Following are some examples of typical x-ray findings per diagnosis:

RHEUMATOID ARTHRITIS

- Tissue changes on both sides of the joint include periarticular swelling, especially of small joints: wrist, MCP, PIP, MTP, and atlantoaxial (AA) joint
- Marginal bone erosion (the disappearance of bone due to pressure)
- Sclerosis (tissue hardening, defined as an attempt by the body to replace structural strength removed by a pathological process)
- No osteophytes
- Minimal or absent reparative processes
- Uniform joint space narrowing
- Rarefaction (lesions) of periarticular regions in the early stages, generalized osteoporosis in the latter stages
- Joint deformities (dislocations)

OSTEOARTHRITIS

- Tissue changes include nonuniform joint space narrowing
- Subchondral bone sclerosis and subarticular cysts
- Osteophyte formation at the joint margins (horizontal bony overgrowth)
- Not bilateral
- Common on DIP (Heberden's nodes), PIP (Bouchard's nodes), CMC, hips, and knees

OSTEOPOROSIS

- Periarticular bone rarefaction (bones become porous or less dense due to absorption of minerals)
- Loss of cortical bone thickness

- Osteopenia (radiographic term for increased bone radiolucency or rarefaction)
- Fractures (spine, wrist, femur, and humerus)

INFECTIONS

- These are characterized radiographically by soft tissue swelling and loss of fat fascial planes. Examples: osteomyelitis, cellulitis, infectious arthritis

BONE TUMORS

- The features for identifying tumors include the site of the lesion
- The fact that they do not cross the joint space
- The type of destruction
- Presence of soft tissue extension of the lesion
- It is rare to have primary bone tumors, and these are mostly seen in children
- Metastases are more common in adults

GOUT

- Bone erosion due to tophus with increased swelling
- Lumps and bumps
- Multiple overhanging margins, especially DIP, first MTT, and elbow
- Decreased joint space

PSORIASIS

- Similar to RA but asymmetrical
- Mostly on DIP with sausage-like appearance, IPJ of toes, SIJ, and spine
- No osteoporosis
- Bone resorption
- Asymmetrical syndesmophytes (vertical "spurs")
- Decreased joint space

ANKYLOSING SPONDYLITIS (AS)

- Calcification of the interspinous ligament, known as "dagger sign"
- Syndesmophytes
- "Bamboo" spine
- Joint space is preserved
- Usually begins at both SI joints
- Ligaments calcify
- Osteoporosis
- "Whiskering" at muscle attachments

CALCIUM PYROPHOSPHATE DIHYDRATE (CPPD)

CPPD crystal deposition is a degenerative arthropathy, not rheumatic, that destroys cartilage. It is similar to osteoarthritis in that it is usually symmetrical with chondrocalcinosis (calcification of cartilage) and rarefaction. Calcium deposits occur in articular cartilage (hyaline or fibrocartilage) and may or may not cause symptoms. It occurs in 4% of adults, but 50% of people above the age of 90 have it. It can be hereditary, idiopathic, traumatic, or due to metabolic diseases (hemochromatosis, thyroid, gout, etc). It has predilection for the first MTT joint and is thus also termed pseudogout. The crystals also deposit in the triangular fibrocartilaginous complex (TFCC) of the wrist, in the elbow, and in the knee, particularly in the patellar area. Symptoms consist of stiffness and achiness, fatigue, and flexion contractures. Due to this and its symmetry, it can easily be confused with RA. In the spine, it can lead to degenerative joint disease and cause cord compression due to hypertrophy of the ligamentum flavum. The treatment consists of colchicine, anti-inflammatories, and surgery to remove the crystals.

DIFFUSE IDIOPATHIC SKELETAL HYPEROSTOSIS (DISH)

DISH or Forestier disease is a calcification of the ligaments, especially the anterior longitudinal ligament of the spine. There is also the development of spurs that form a bony bridge in at least four vertebrae on the anterolateral aspect of the vertebral body without degenerative disc disease or osteoporosis, so the vertebral space is relatively preserved. Unlike ankylosing spondylitis, there is minimal to no sacroiliac joint involvement. DISH affects white males more than females older than the age of 65, especially if overweight. Its etiology is unknown, but there is a link to diabetes, obesity, and HLA-B27. The disease can progress to other joints, especially to the knee, medial epicondyle, and the Achilles' tendon. It may coexist with RA and gout.

HETEROTOPIC OSSIFICATION (HO)

HO is an osteoblastic activity (versus a calcium deposition) that usually occurs after prolonged immobilization. It is seen frequently in patients with traumatic brain injury (TBI), spinal cord injury (SCI), and total hip replacement (THR). Unlike calcific tendinitis or myositis ossificans, there is actual trabecular bone within the ossification.

RADIOGRAPHIC MEASUREMENTS

Studies have been performed detailing normal values for angles, ratios, and distances between certain joints. These norms help the clinician assess whether there are deficits in alignment, and they give a baseline to determine whether a particular intervention may be effective or not. It also helps determine if there are contraindications to movement (eg, spurs that may cause bony blocks into rotation of the spine).

These measurements are also known as lines of mensuration. Some of the most common lines include the following:

UPPER EXTREMITY

- *Acromiohumeral distance:* This distance is measured on an A-P film of the shoulder in neutral. The normal interval between the humeral head and the inferior portion of the acromion is 7 to 14 mm. Narrowing of 5 mm or less is abnormal (Figure 13-1).

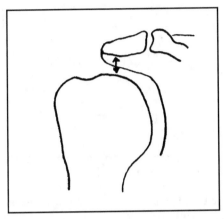

Figure 13-1. Acromiohumeral distance.

- *Ulnar variance:* This is measured on an A-P film and normally, the distal ulna and the distal radius are level. It is a line extended from the distal radial articular surface toward the ulna, and the distance from this line to the distal ulna is measured in millimeters. A short ulna is termed negative variance (Figure 13-2).

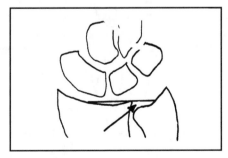

Figure 13-2. Ulnar variance.

- *Wrist arcs:* These are three arcuate lines drawn on a neutral A-P film along the proximal margins of the scaphoid, lunate, triquetrum, distal margins of the same bones, and the proximal margins of the capitate and hamate. These arcs of Gilula should normally be smooth. Note the cartilage spaces. The distances between the carpal bones is normally even throughout the wrist. Widening, especially at the scapholunate joint, between 2 and 4 mm is abnormal (Figure 13-3).

Figure 13-3. Wrist arcs.

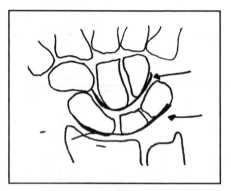

- *Capitolunate angle:* This is measured on a lateral film with two lines drawn bisecting the capitate and the lunate on their longitudinal axes. The angle of intersection of the two lines should be 0 degrees. If greater than 20 degrees, it is abnormal (Figure 13-4).

Figure 13-4. Capitolunate angle.

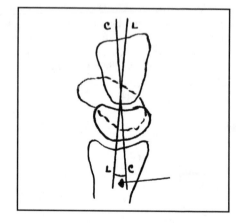

- *Scapholunate angle*: Similar to the capitolunate angle, the lines bisecting the longitudinal axes of the scaphoid and lunate should normally be 30 to 60 degrees. In normal hands, the longitudinal axes of the radius, lunate, capitate, and third metacarpal are collinear. The scapholunate angle formed by the longitudinal axes of each bone averages 46 degrees. If the scaphoid is more dorsal, it is a dorsal intercalated segmental instability (DISI) lesion (Figure 13-5).

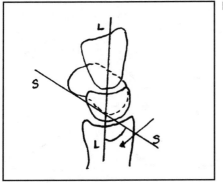

Figure 13-5. Scapholunate angle.

SPINE

- *Alignment:* On a lateral film and throughout the spine starting from C2 down, there should be smooth and unbroken arcs—one on the anterior margins of the vertebral bodies, one on the posterior margins, and one through the spinous processes. There are also soft tissue spaces that must be aligned on a normal neck: the retropharyngeal space of < 5 mm (from C3 anteriorly to the first shadow) and the retrolaryngeal space of < 22 mm (from C6 to the first shadow) (Figure 13-6).

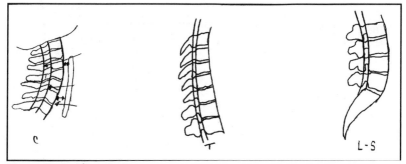

Figure 13-6. Alignment.

- *Cobb's method for scoliosis:* Two lines are drawn along the superior and inferior endplates of the upper and lower vertebrae, respectively, which tilt maximally toward the concavity of the curve (end vertebra). It may be necessary to construct perpendiculars to these lines for technical reasons to measure lesser angles on the film (Figure 13-7).

Figure 13-7. Cobb's method for scoliosis.

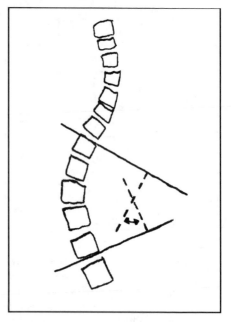

- *Rotational deformity:* Vertical rotation is assessed by observing the symmetry between the pedicles and the lateral borders of the body on an A-P film. As rotation occurs, the pedicle on the convex side is displaced further from the lateral edge of the vertebra toward the midline (Figure 13-8).

Figure 13-8. Rotational deformity.

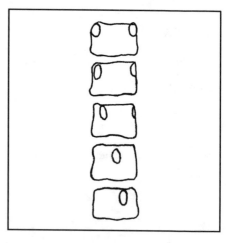

- *Atlas-odontoid distance:* This is measured on a lateral film with the head and neck in neutral. The distance between the posterior inferior margin of the anterior arch of the atlas and the anterior surface of the dens is measured. The maximum displacement in a normal child is 5 mm, and in adults, it is between 2 and 4 mm (Figure 13-9).

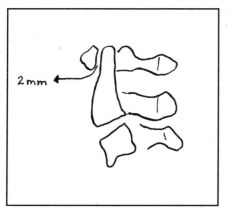

Figure 13-9. Atlas-odontoid distance.

- *Sacral and lumbosacral angle:* A normal angle of 30 degrees is measured by drawing a horizontal line on a lateral film and intersecting it with a line drawn on the superior surface of S1. The lumbosacral angle is between the lumbar spine and sacrum with its apex at L5 disc space. Normal value is 140 degrees (Figure 13-10).

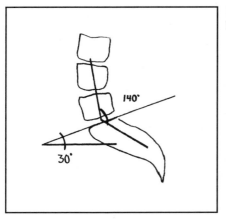

Figure 13-10. Sacral and lumbosacral angle.

LOWER EXTREMITY

- *Shenton's line:* This curve is drawn from the medial curve of the edge of the femur to the inferior edge of the pubis. If this arc is broken, it may indicate a fracture or dislocation (Figure 13-11).

Figure 13-11. Shenton's line.

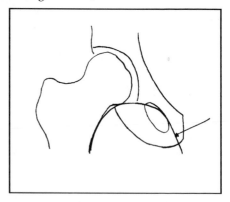

- *Angle of inclination:* A normal angle of 125 degrees is formed by the angle between the neck and the shaft of the femur to show coxa vara or valga (Figure 13-12).

Figure 13-12. Angle of inclination.

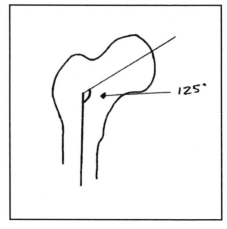

- *Q-angle:* This is the angle formed by the rectus femoris muscle and the patellar tendon. It helps assess problems like patellofemoral pain syndrome, femoral anteversion, valgus, and subluxing patella among others. It is formed by intersecting a line from the ASIS to the center of the patella and a line from the tibial tubercle to the center of the patella, with the hip in neutral. Normally, the line is 13 degrees in men and 18 degrees in women (Figure 13-13).

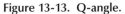

Figure 13-13. Q-angle.

- *Index of Insall and Salvati:* This assesses the position of the patella and is the ratio between the length of the patellar tendon and the length of the patella measured on a lateral film, usually at 30 degrees of knee flexion. The height of the patella is measured from its proximal posterior border to the distal pole. The patellar tendon is measured from its proximal posterior attachment, immediately above the apex of the patella, to the notch on the proximal margin of the tibial tubercle. Normally, the ratio is relatively even and does not exceed 20%. If greater than 20%, then there is patella alta (Figure 13-14).

Figure 13-14. Index of Insall and Salvati.

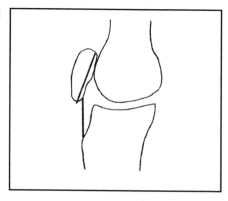

- *Sulcus angle:* This is measured on a tangential or sunrise view of the knee and is normally 138 degrees ±6 degrees. The angle is formed by the highest points of the medial and lateral femoral condyles and the lowest point of the intercondylar sulcus. If shallow, it is related to patellar dislocations (Figure 13-15).

Figure 13-15. Sulcus angle.

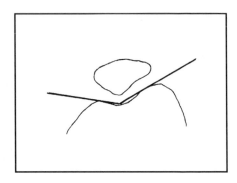

- *Lateral patellar displacement*: A line is drawn on the highest points of the medial and lateral femoral condyles. A perpendicular line is then drawn to that line at the medial edge of the medial condyle, and the last line is drawn at the edge of the lateral patella. The distance between these two lines should be less than 1 mm (Figure 13-16).

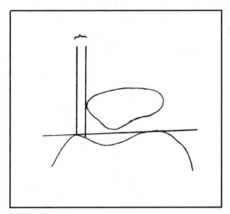

Figure 13-16. Lateral patellar displacement.

- *Lateral patellofemoral angle:* This is the angle of intersection between a line connecting the apices of the femoral condyles and a line drawn along the lateral femoral surface. This usually opens laterally or, rarely, is parallel. In patients with subluxation, the line may be parallel or open medially (Figure 13-17).

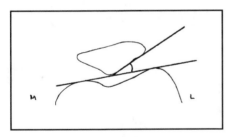

Figure 13-17. Lateral patellarofemoral angle.

- *Talar tilt:* This angle is measured on a stress film with the ankle inverted. A line is drawn on the inferior surface of the tibia and on the superior surface on the talus. The intersection is the angle of talar tilt. Also, assess the distance from the medial malleolus to the talus. The normal clear space is of 2 to 3 mm width. A normal tilt averages 7 degrees, but it should be compared bilaterally because of the wide range of variability. A tilt of 35 degrees can denote a complete ligamentous rupture (Figure 13-18).

Figure 13-18. Talar tilt.

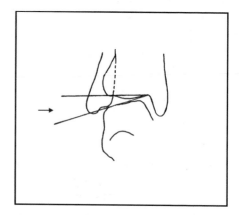

- *Böhler's angle:* On a lateral ankle film, this is measured by drawing a line between the posterior superior aspect of the calcaneus and the highest point of the posterior subtalar articular surface. Normally, the angle is 30 to 35 degrees. A decrease in the angle denotes a subtalar joint problem, usually a fracture (Figure 13-19).

Figure 13-19. Böhler's angle.

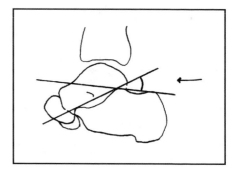

BIBLIOGRAPHY

Anderson M, Hall S. *Fundamentals of Sports Injury Management*. Baltimore, Md: Williams & Wilkins; 1997.

Bahr R, Pena F, Shine J, Lew W, Tyrdal S, Engebretsen L. Biomechanics of ankle ligament reconstruction. An invitro comparison of the Brostrom repair, Watson-Jones reconstruction, and a new anatomic reconstruction technique. *Am J Sports Med*. 1997;25(4):424-432.

Benson E, Schutzer S. Posttraumatic piriformis syndrome: diagnosis and results of operative treatment. *Bone Joint Surg*. 1999;81-A(7):941-949.

Berg E, Ciullo J. A clinical test for superior glenoid labral or "SLAP" lesions. *Clinical Journal of Sports Medicine*. 1998;8(2):121-123.

Bogduk N. *Clinical Anatomy of the Lumbar Spine*. New York, NY: Churchill Livingstone; 1997.

Brotzman B. *Clinical Orthopaedic Rehabilitation*. St. Louis, Mo: Mosby; 1996.

Corso G. Impingement relief test: an adjunctive procedure to traditional assessment of shoulder impingement syndrome. *Phys Ther*. 1995;22(5):183-192.

Cortet B, Boutry N, Flipo R, Duquesnoy B, Chastanet P, Delcambre B. Percutaneous vertebroplasty in the treatment of compression fractures: an open prospective study. *J Rheumatol*. 1999;26(10):2222-2228.

DeFranca G, Levine L. T-4 syndrome. *J Manipulative Physiol Ther*. 1995;18(1):34-37.

Di Fabio R. Disablement: the patient's problem no longer matters. *JOSPT*. 2000;30(6): 304-305.

Donatelli R. *The Biomechanics of the Foot and Ankle*. Philadelphia, Pa: FA Davis; 1990.

Donatelli R, Wooden M. *Orthopaedic Physical Therapy*. New York, NY: Churchill Livingstone; 1989.

Donelson R, Aprill C, Medcalf R, Grant W. A prospective study of centralization of the lumbar spine and referred pain. *Spine*. 1997;22(10):1115-1122.

Elliot BG. Finkelstein test: a descriptive error that can cause a false positive. *J Hand Surg*. 1992;17B(4):481-482.

Evans R. *Illustrated Essentials in Orthopaedic Physical Assessment*. St. Louis, Mo: Mosby; 1994.

Fehlandt A, Micheli L. Acute exertional compartment syndrome in an adolescent female. *Med Sci Sports Exerc*. 1995;27(1):3-7.

Gehlsen G, Ganion L, Helfst R. Fibroblast responses to variations in soft tissue mobilization. *Med Sci Sports Exerc*. 1999;31(4):531-535.

Glynn C, Crockford G, Gavaghan D, Cardno P, Price O, Miller J. Epidemiology of shingles. *JR Soc Med*. 1990;83(10):617-619.

Gray J. Diagnosis of intermittent vascular claudication in a patient with diagnosis of sciatica. *Phys Ther*. 1999;79(6):582-590.

Greenman P. *Principles of Manual Medicine*. 2nd ed. Baltimore, Md: Williams and Wilkins; 1996.

Greenwood M, Erhard R, Jones D. Differential diagnosis of the hip vs. lumbar spine: Five case reports. *JOSPT*. 1998;27(4):308-315.

Grelsamer R, McConnell J. *The Patella*. Gaithersburg, Md: Aspen Publishers; 1998.

Hall C, Brody L. *Therapeutic Exercise: Moving Toward Function*. Philadelphia, Pa: Lippincott, Williams & Wilkins; 1999.

Halle JS, Franklin R, Karalfa B. Comparison of four treatment approaches for lateral epicondylitis of the elbow. *JOSPT*. 1986;8(2):62-68.

Hase T, Ueo T. Acetabular labral tear: arthroscopic diagnosis and treatment. *Arthroscopy*. 1999;15(2):138-141.

Hertling D, Kessler R. *Management of Common Musculoskeletal Disorders: Physical Therapy Principles and Methods*. 3rd ed. Philadelphia, Pa: Lippincott; 1996.

Itoi E, Kido T, Sano A, Urayama M, Sato K. Which is more useful, the "full can test" or the "empty can test" in detecting the torn supraspinatus tendon? *Am J Sports Med*. 1999;27(1):65-68.

Jones DM. Radiographic abnormalities of the lumbar spine in college football players. *Am J Sports Med*. 1999;27(3):335-338.

Kisner C, Colby L. *Therapeutic Exercise: Foundations and Techniques*. 3rd ed. Philadelphia, Pa: FA Davis; 1996.

Klippel J, ed. *Primer on the Rheumatic Diseases*. 11th ed. Atlanta, Ga: Arthritis Foundation; 1997.

Kopp J, Alexander H, Turocy R, Levrini M, Lichtman D. The use of lumbar extension in the evaluation and treatment of patients with acute herniated nucleus pulposus. A preliminary report. *Clin Orthop*. 1984;202: 211-218.

Kuhlman K, Hennessey D, Hennessey M. Sensitivity and specificity of carpal tunnel syndrome signs. *Am J Phys Med Rehabil*. 1997;76:451-457.

Loth T, Wadsworth C. *Orthopedic Review for Physical Therapists*. St. Louis, Mo: Mosby; 1998.

Magee D. *Orthopaedic Physical Assessment*. 3rd ed. Philadelphia, Pa: WB Saunders; 1997.

Malone T, McPoil T, Nitz A. *Orthopedic and Sports Physical Therapy*. 3rd ed. St. Louis, Mo: Mosby; 1997.

Mata S, Fortin P, Fitzcharles M, et al. A controlled study of diffuse idiopathic skeletal hyperostosis. Clinical features and functional status. *Medicine*. 1997;76:104-117.

McCarty E, Tsairis P, Warren R. Brachial neuritis. *Clin Orthop*. 1999;368: 37-43.

McKenzie R. *The Lumbar Spine: Mechanical Diagnosis and Therapy*. New Zealand: Spinal Publications, Ltd; 1981.

McKinnis L. *Fundamentals of Orthopaedic Radiology*. Philadelphia, Pa: FA Davis; 1997.

Mimori K. A new pain provocation test for superior labral tears of the shoulder. *Am J Sports Med*. 1999;27(3):137-142.

Mortensen N, Skov O, Jensen P. Early motion of the ankle after operative treatment of a rupture of the Achilles' tendon. A prospective, randomized clinical and radiographic study. *J Bone Joint Surg*. 1999;81-A (7):983-990.

Motley G, Nyland J, Jacobs J, Caborn D. The pars interarticularis stress reaction, spondylolysis, spondylolisthesis progression. *Journal of Athletic Training*. 1998;33(4):351-358.

Park W, Hughes S, eds. *Orthopaedic Radiology*. Oxford: Blackwell Scientific Publications; 1987.

Probe R, Baca M, Adams R, Preece C. Night splint treatment for plantar fasciitis. A prospective, randomized study. *Clin Orthop*. 1999;(368):190-195.

Rachlin E. *Myofascial Pain and Fibromyalgia: Trigger Point Management*. St. Louis, Mo: Mosby; 1994.

Roy S, Irvin R. *Sports Medicine: Prevention, Evaluation, Management, and Rehabilitation*. Englewood Cliffs, NJ: Prentice Hall; 1983.

Saunders HD, Saunders R. *Evaluation, Treatment, and Prevention of Musculoskeletal Disorders. Vol. 1, Spine*. Bloomington, Ind: Saunders & Saunders; 1993.

Shelbourne D, Nitz P. Accelerated rehabilitation after anterior cruciate ligament reconstruction. *JOSPT*. 1992;15(6):256-264.

Shinabarger N. Limited joint mobility in adults with diabetes mellitus. *Phys Ther*. 1987;67(2):215-218.

Slater R. *Textbook of Disorders and Injuries of the Musculoskeletal System*. 3rd ed. Baltimore, Md: Williams & Wilkins; 1999.

Sobel J, Sollenberger P, Robinson R, Polatin P, Gatchel R. Cervical non-organic signs: a new clinical tool to assess abnormal illness behavior in neck pain patients. A pilot study. *Arch Phys Med Rehabil*. 2000;81:170-175.

Stanley B, Tribuzi S. *Concepts in Hand Rehabilitation*. Philadelphia, Pa: FA Davis; 1992.

Tetro M, Evanoff S, Hollstein S, Gelberman R. A new provocation test for carpal tunnel syndrome. *JBJS*. 1998;80B(3):493-498.

Ubachs J, Slooff A, Peeters L. Obstetric antecedents of surgically treated obstetric brachial plexus injuries. *Br J Obstet Gynaecol*. 1995;102(10):813-817.

Waddell G, McCulloch J, Kummel E, Venner R. Nonorganic physical signs in low back pain. *Spine*. 1981;5:117-125.

Wadsworth C. Peripheral nerve compression neuropathy. La Crosse, Wis: *Orthopaedic Physical Therapy Home Study Course: The Elbow, Forearm and Wrist*. 1997.

Waggy C. Disorders of the wrist. La Crosse, Wis: *Orthopaedic Physical Therapy Home Study Course: The Elbow, Forearm and Wrist*. 1997.

Weissman B, Sledge C, Clement B. *Orthopaedic Radiology*. Philadelphia, Pa: WB Saunders; 1986.

Winkle D. *Diagnosis and Treatment of the Spine*. Gaithersburg, Md: Aspen Publishers; 1996.

APPENDICES

APPENDIX A

CAPSULAR PATTERNS AND JOINT POSITIONS

Joint	Capsular Pattern	Open Pack Position	Closed Pack Position
Glenohumeral	External rotation, abduction, internal rotation	55-degree flexion, 30-degree horizontal abduction	External rotation, abduction
Sternoclavicular	Pain at end ranges	Arm resting at the side	Full shoulder elevation
Acromioclavicular	Pain at end ranges	Arm resting at the side	90-degree abduction
Ulnohumeral	Flexion, extension	70-degree flexion, 10-degree supination	Extension
Radiohumeral	Flexion, extension, supination, pronation	Extension, supination	90-degree flexion, 5-degree supination
Proximal radio-ulnar	Supination, pronation	70-degree flexion, 35-degree supination	5-degree supination
Distal radioulnar	Pain with full rotation	10-degree supination	5-degree supination
Wrist	Flexion and extension equally limited	Neutral with slight ulnar deviation	Extension with radial deviation
Trapeziometa-carpal	Abduction, extension	Neutral	Opposition
Metacarpo-phalangeal	Flexion, extension	Slight extension	Flexion
Interphalangeal	Flexion, extension	Slight flexion	Extension
Temporo-mandibular	Opening	Slight opening	Closing
Occipitoatlantal	Extension and side-bending equally limited	Neutral between flexion and extension	Extension
Cervical spine	Side-bending and rotation equally limited, extension	Neutral between flexion and extension	Extension

Appendix A (continued)

Capsular Patterns and Joint Positions

Joint	Capsular Pattern	Open Pack Position	Closed Pack Position
Thoracic spine	Side-bending and rotation equally limited, extension	Neutral between flexion and extension	Extension
Lumbar spine	Side-bending and rotation equally limited, extension	Neutral between flexion and extension	Extension
Sacroiliac	Pain with joint stress	N/A	N/A
Hip	Flexion, abduction, internal rotation (order can change)	30-degree flexion, 30-degree abduction, slight external rotation	Extension, internal rotation, abduction
Knee	Flexion, extension	25-degree flexion	Extension, tibia external rotation
Tibiofibular	Pain with joint stress	N/A	N/A
Talocrural	Plantarflexion, dorsiflexion	10-degree plantarflexion	Dorsiflexion
Subtalar	Inversion	Neutral	Supination
Midtarsal	Dorsiflexion, plantarflexion, adduction, internal rotation	Neutral	Supination
Great toe	Extension, flexion	Neutral	Extension
Second to fifth metatarsophalangeal	Varies	Neutral	Extension
Interphalangeal	Flexion, extension	Slight flexion	Extension

APPENDIX B

END FEELS			
End Feel	*Type*	*Description*	*Example*
Bone-to-bone	Normal	Pain-free, hard, and unyielding feeling	Elbow extension
Soft tissue approximation	Normal	Gradual soft yielding due to compression of soft tissue	Elbow and knee flexion
Tissue stretch	Normal	Firm resistance with slight yielding due to tightness	Shoulder— external rotation, ankle dorsiflexion
Muscle spasm	Abnormal	Sudden limitation of motion with pain	Upper trazpezius hypertonicity
Capsular	Abnormal	Firm resistance through the range with slight yielding in unexpected areas, can be soft or hard	Soft: ankle sprain Hard: frozen shoulder
Bone-to-bone	Abnormal	Hard, unyielding sensation before the end of the range	Cervical rotation limited by spurs
Empty	Abnormal	Pain stops the motion, not other tissues	Acute bursitis
Springy block	Abnormal	Rebound sensation with firm resistance and tightness in unexpected areas	Meniscal injury, blocking motion

APPENDIX C

WADDELL'S NONORGANIC PHYSICAL SIGNS

A. Subjective Symptoms

1. Have you ever had whole leg pain?
   - pos.   neg.
2. Have you ever had whole leg numbness?
   - pos.   neg.
3. Has your whole leg ever given away?
   - pos.   neg.
4. Has there ever been a period of time with very little pain?
   - pos.   neg.
5. Have you ever been unable to tolerate therapy because of pain?
   - pos.   neg.
6. Have you ever had pain on the tip of your tail bone?
   - pos.   neg.
7. Have you ever been admitted to the ER due to pain?
   - pos.   neg.

B. Objective Signs

1. Axial loading	pos.	neg.
2. Simulated trunk rotation	pos.	neg.
3. Exaggerated pain behaviors during testing	pos.	neg.
4. Superficial tenderness on the lumbar spine	pos.	neg.
5. Distracted SLR supine versus sitting	pos.	neg.
6. Nonanatomical sensory dermatome	pos.	neg.
7. Nonanatomical motor myotome	pos.	neg.

Score of positives _____

Interpretation

0 to 2—negative magnified illness behavior
2 to 5—minimal magnified illness behavior
5 to 7—moderate magnified illness behavior
7 to 14—maximum magnified illness behavior

INDEX

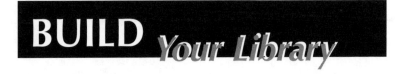

BUILD Your Library

This book and many others on numerous different topics are available from SLACK Incorporated. For further information or a copy of our latest catalog, contact us at:

Professional Book Division
SLACK Incorporated
6900 Grove Road
Thorofare, NJ 08086 USA
Telephone: 1-856-848-1000
1-800-257-8290
Fax: 1-856-853-5991
E-mail: orders@slackinc.com
www.slackbooks.com

We accept most major credit cards and checks or money orders in US dollars drawn on a US bank. Most orders are shipped within 72 hours.

Contact us for information on recent releases, forthcoming titles, and bestsellers. If you have a comment about this title or see a need for a new book, direct your correspondence to the Editorial Director at the above address.

Thank you for your interest and we hope you found this work beneficial.